ADVICES TO DIABETIC PATIENTS

HOW TO AVOID THE LOSS OF A LEG

Dr. Enrique Uguet, Ph. D.

I0480273

ADVICES TO DIABETIC PATIENTS. HOW TO AVOID THE LOSS OF A LEG?

Professor Dr. Enrique Uguet, PHD.
Physician Surgeon Specialist in
Angiology and Vascular Surgery. Cuba.
Doctor in Philosophy in
Biomedical Sciences

Advice to Diabetic Patients.
How to avoid the loss of a leg?

First edition 2017

Design and composition edition: The author

Cover design: The author

Photographs: Author's property.

Drawings: Pages:4, 25, 26, 27, 29, 30, 32, 33, 34, 35, 36, 37, 38, 39, 40, 41, 42, 43, 48, 50, 53, 55, 58, 59, 61. 62. 63. 64, 65, 67, 69, 71, 72, 77, 87, 94, 95, 96 y 98, Alex Cardoso. Master in Arts in Graphic Design.

Rest of the drawings: The author

ISBN: B&W 10: 1974270068

(B&W) 13: 9781974270064

I want to thank for the help I have received in the

translation from Spanish to English of this book to:

Mr. Jose Páez. Bachelor of Art in Philosophy.

Bachelor of Art in Political Science.

Mr. Enrique Martínez. Bachelor of Art in Digital Media-Game Design.

To all diabetic patients I have dealt with a complication in their lower limbs and to their relatives who relied on me to restore their health. Both can live in peace because I made available to them all my physical and intellectual capacity that I possessed to give them the best solution to their problems.

INTRODUCTION

Dear diabetic patient, the purpose of this book is:

1. To alert yourself about the real possibility you may have of suffering an amputation in your legs.

2. To explain in a scientific way, understandable and enjoyable, the characteristics of complications that can manifest in your feet.

3. Recommend an organized and logical method for you to examine your feet daily.

4. And give you the fundamental advice about the behavior you must follow to prevent complications and to avoid these possible consequences from causing you to change your lifestyle.

You cannot consider the possibility of an unfavorable evolution as something against which it is not possible to fight. It is proven that the incidence of amputations in the diabetic can be reduced, delayed or avoided if you spend some time of the day educating yourself about the misfortunes that lurk at your feet, but it is not only illustrate and know when to detect the dangerous characteristics which indicate a potential risk for their full preservation, but to assist the primary care physician promptly and be attended, if necessary, by a specialist.

It is not convenient to feel rooted in the routine of daily life, you need to make an intellectual change that is offered to you in this set of pages, which you should hold on to and be captivated with to develop your cultural and manuals skills in order to understand the causes that govern the negative anatomical events that prowl at your feet, and act with the hope and skill necessary to achieve the purposes that this publication aims: to prevent the amputation of a limb.

It is enough for you to open the pages, to penetrate in its content, so that you feel circulating in your brain a feeling of benefactor learning. Your life should consist of filling your neurons with knowledge every minute you devote to your reading. It is unforgivable that you proceed in contradiction to your own interests, and thus extend your hands and grab this copy as plants seize the environment rich in light and oxygen. You have in your health insurance the Primary Doctor and the Endocrinologist in charge of controlling the evolution of your diabetes, you have the Podologist for the periodic attention of your feet, you can buy the medicines to lower the blood glucose in the pharmacy to which you are affiliated, and the Dietitian must have explained perfectly well, what are the foods, in what quantity and hour you should ingest them.

The rest depends on you, it is necessary that you follow the directions of your doctor and my book very precisely and thus you will have as reward **a longer life, healthy and without amputations**.

Dear diabetic patient, you can have in your legs four types of complications.

1. COMPLICATIONS OF THE ARTERIAL BLOOD CIRCULATION BY REDUCTION OR ABSENCE OF BLOOD (ISCHEMIC).

Lack of blood by occlusion of your arteries that causes a pale or blue coloration.

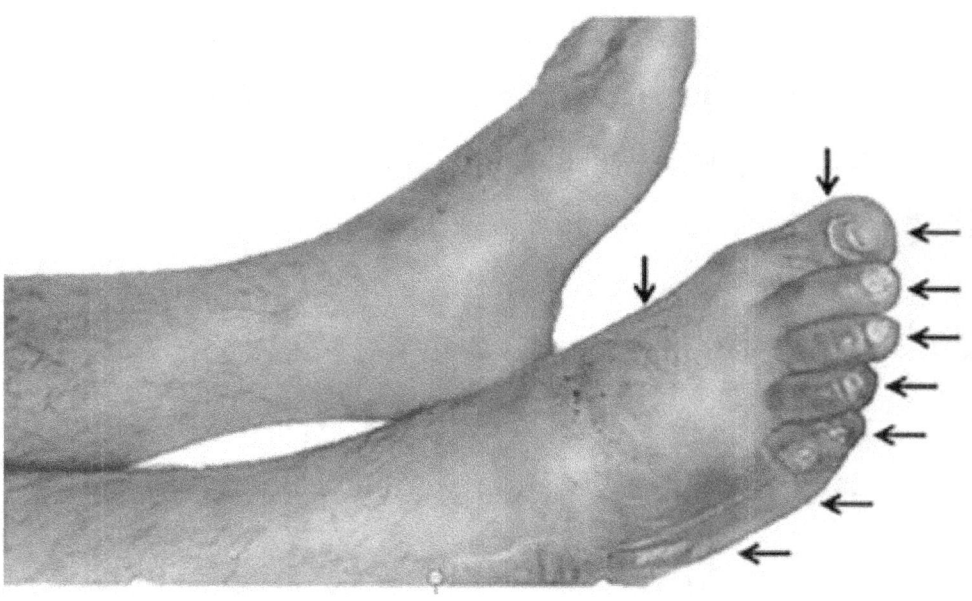

CYANOTIC (BLUE) SPOTTED OF THE RIGHT FOOT

If the lack of blood is important it cause an ulceration.

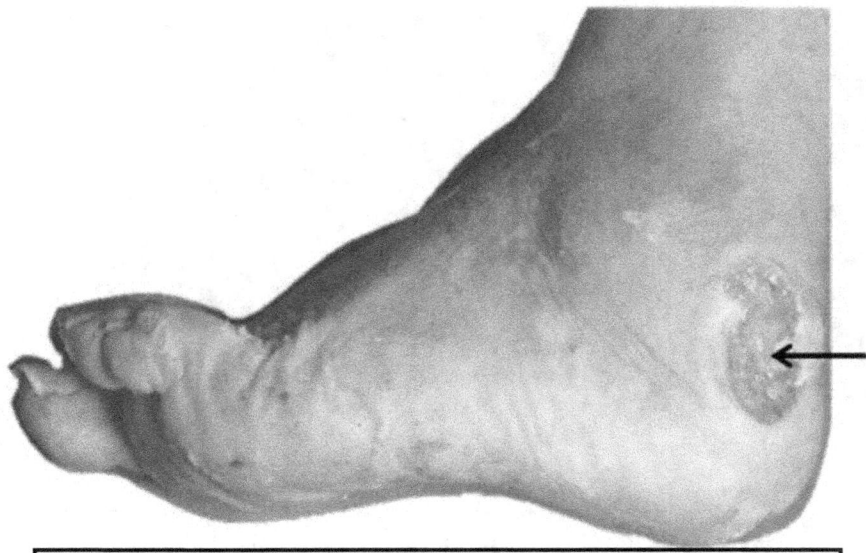

ISCHEMIC ULCER OF THE RIGHT FOOT

When the absence of blood intensifies the tissues

die and is called gangrene.

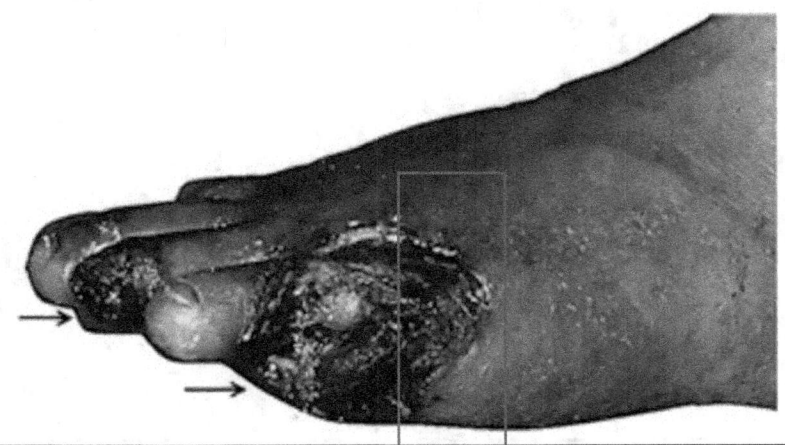

GANGRENA LOCATED IN THE 1st AND 3rd
TOES OF THE RIGHT FOOT

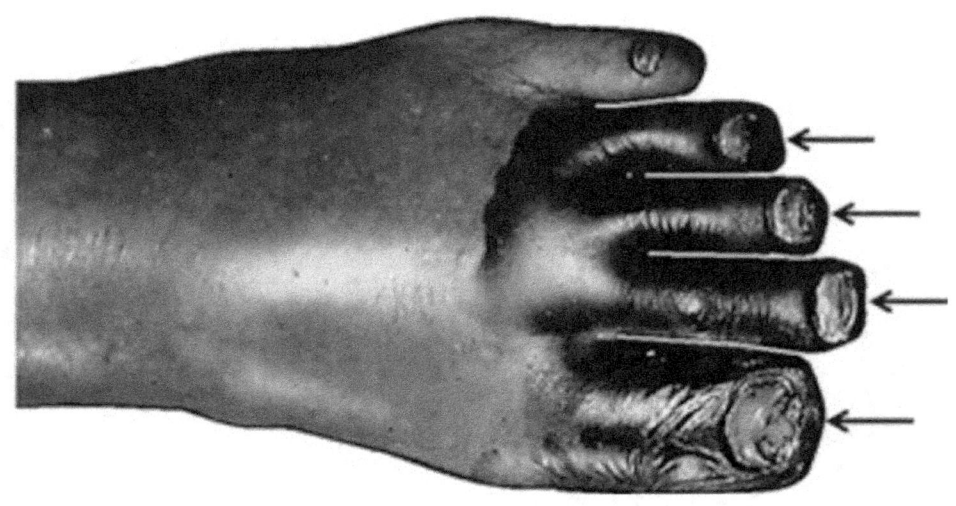

GANGRENE EXTENDING TO FOUR TOES OF LEFT FOOT

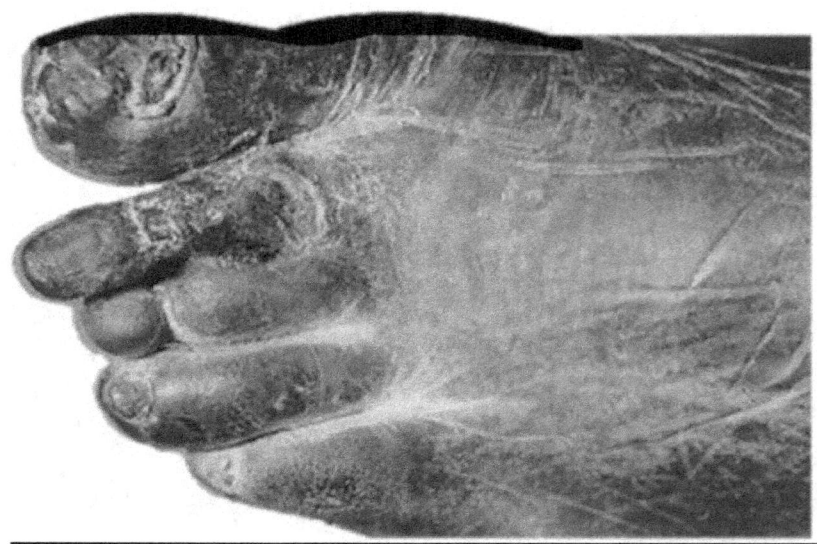

GANGRENE EXTENDING TO THE LEFT FOOT

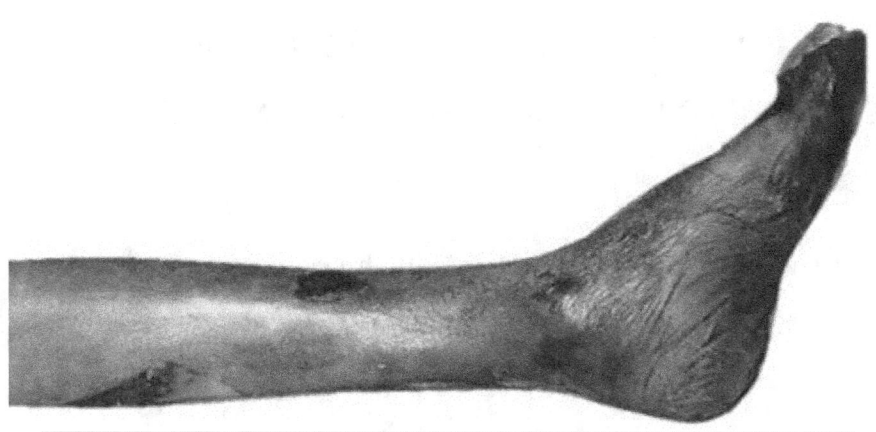

GANGRENE EXTENDING TO THE LEFT FOOT
AND LEG

2. INFECTIOUS COMPLICATIONS FOR PENETRATION AND DEVELOPMENT OF GERMS

They give rise to the formation of abscesses.

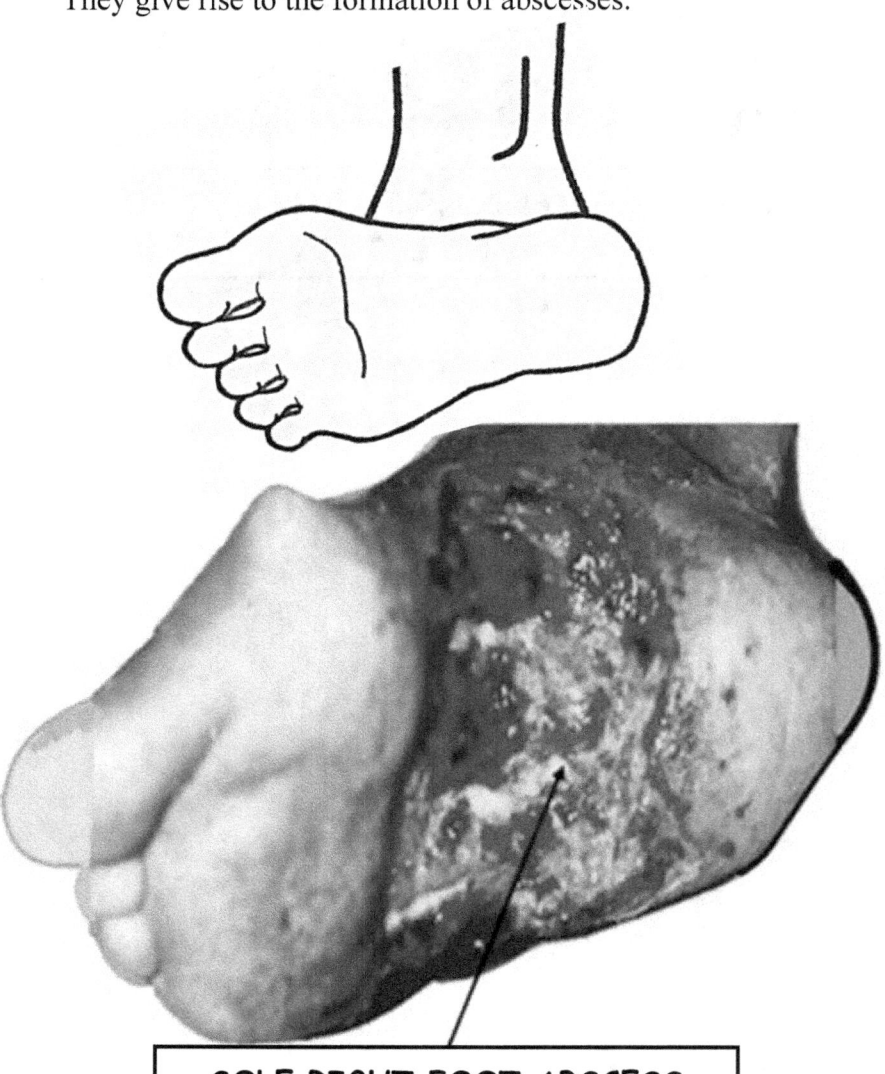

SOLE RIGHT FOOT ABSCESS

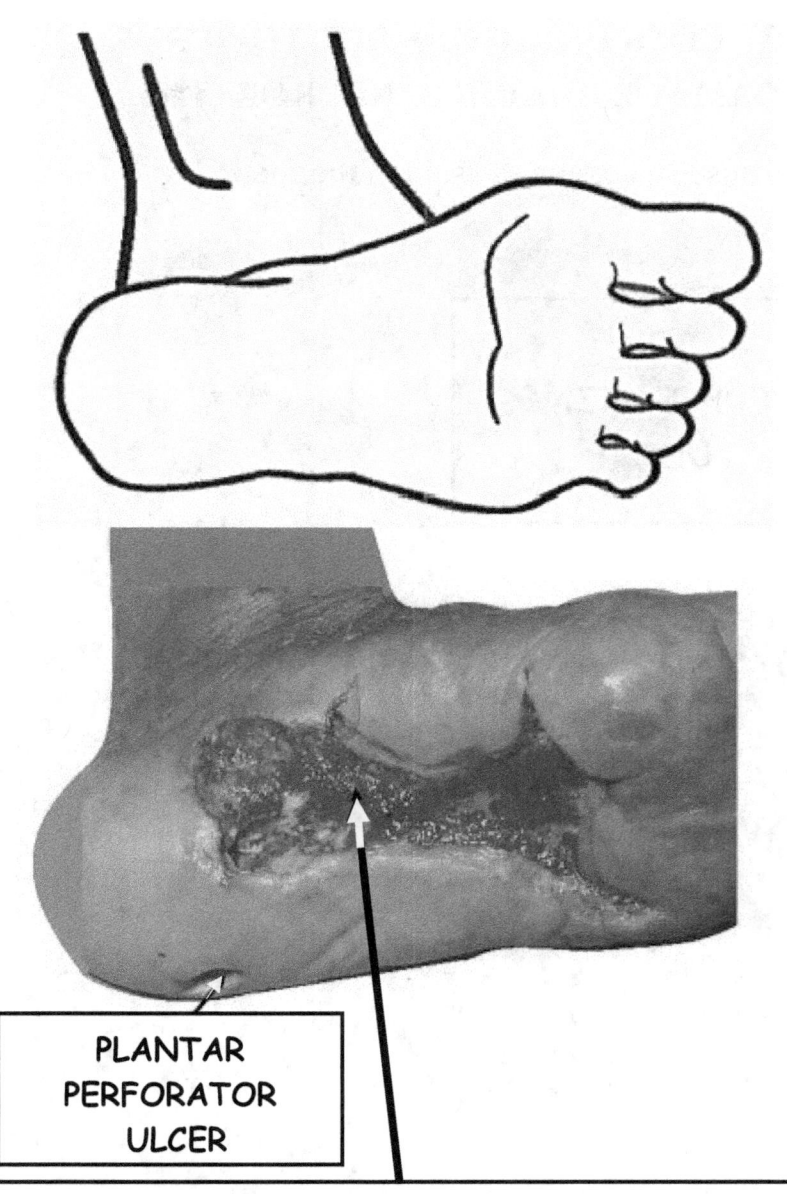

PLANTAR
PERFORATOR
ULCER

LEFT FOOT PLANTAR ABSCESS CUTTED AND
DRAINED.

3. COMPLICATIONS DUE TO NERVE DAMAGE (DIABETIC NEUROPATHY).

Causes ulcers on the sole of the foot.

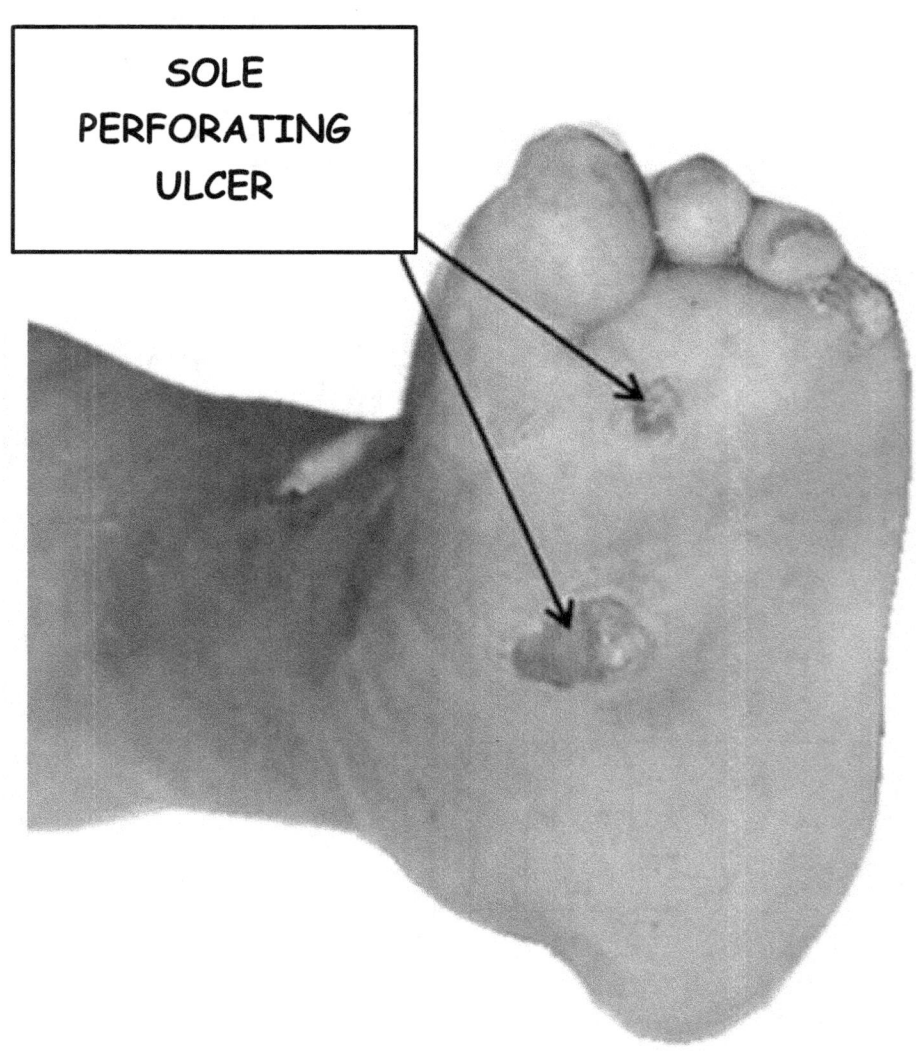

SOLE PERFORATING ULCER

4. JOINTS COMPLICATIONS.
DEFORMITIES.

They also cause ulcers on the sole of the foot that can be the gateway to germs and cause an abscess.

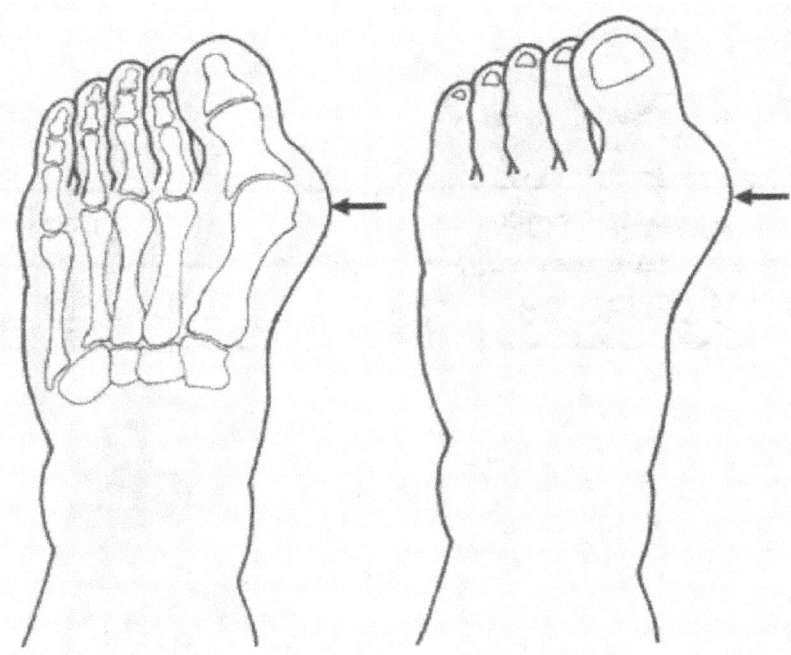

BUNION

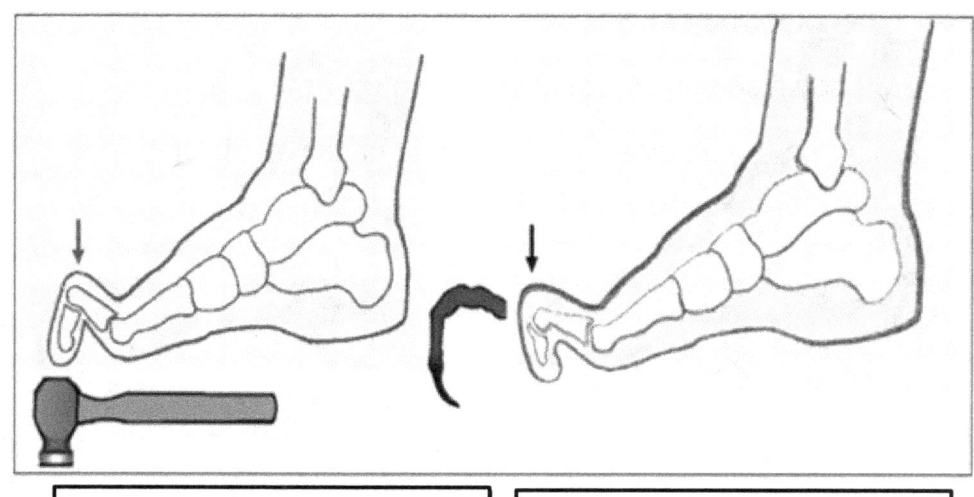

HAMMER TOES	CLAW TOES
FIGURE 18	FIGURE 19

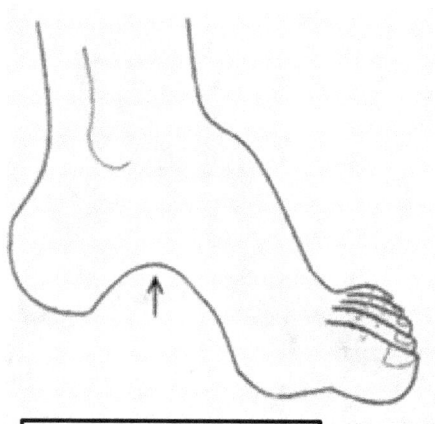

CAVUS FOOT

FIGURE 20

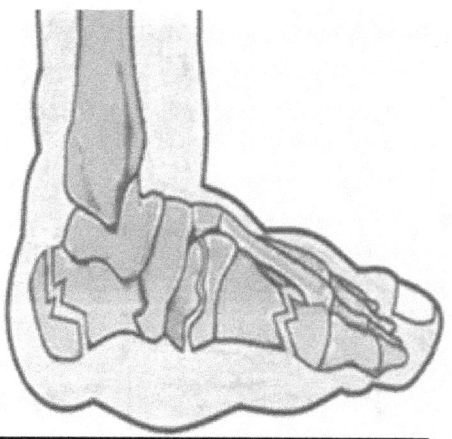

CHARCOT FOOT

FIGURE 21

THE FEET EXAM

The diabetic must have an organized mind and trace a methodological routine to explore his feet, always following the same order, to create a beneficial procedural habit that prevents him from forgetting certain regions of the foot and his goals. Sometimes the mistakes that can be made are not the result of errors in the interpretation of the findings, but by omission in the examination.

To periodically examine your feet:

a) Sit in a place where you are comfortable.

b) Adopt a position to facilitate observation.

c) Select the most appropriate time.

d) Provide excellent lighting.

e) Take the time that is necessary.

f) If you have visual defects and wear glasses, do not forget them.

g) You can be provided yourself with a magnifying glass for more precise observation.

h) Use a large magnifying mirror to look at the plantar region.

i) If you have any impediment to observe your feet, requires the collaboration of a relative or acquaintance.

j) When in doubt about any finding, compare it with the other foot if it is healthy.

The results of these tests will determine your need to consult your primary doctor or podiatrist and the urgency with which you should do so. In the doubt, consult as soon as possible.

ADVICE TO DIABETICS TO AVOID AN AMPUTATION

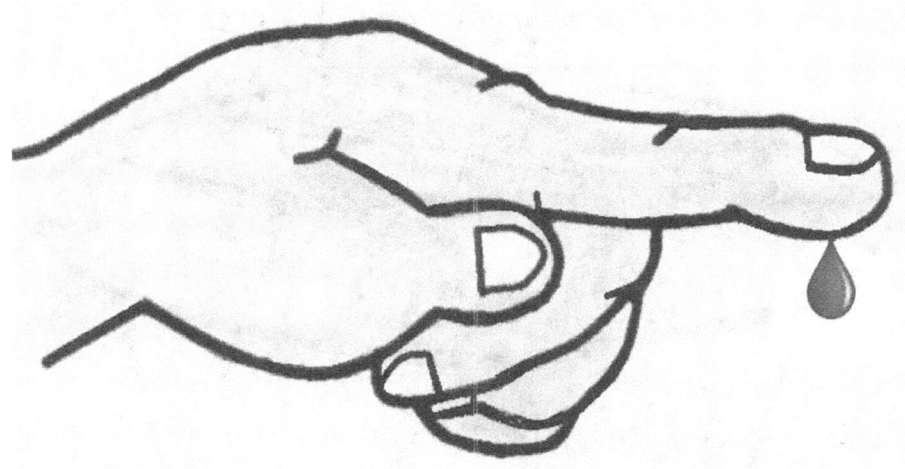

ADVICE #1
CHECK YOUR DIABETES DAILY: FOLLOWING
YOUR DOCTOR'S DRUG TREATMENT,
MEASURING THE SUGAR LEVEL IN THE
BLOOD WITH THE GLUCOMETER AND
EATING THE FOOD RECOMMENDED BY THE
DIETITIAN.

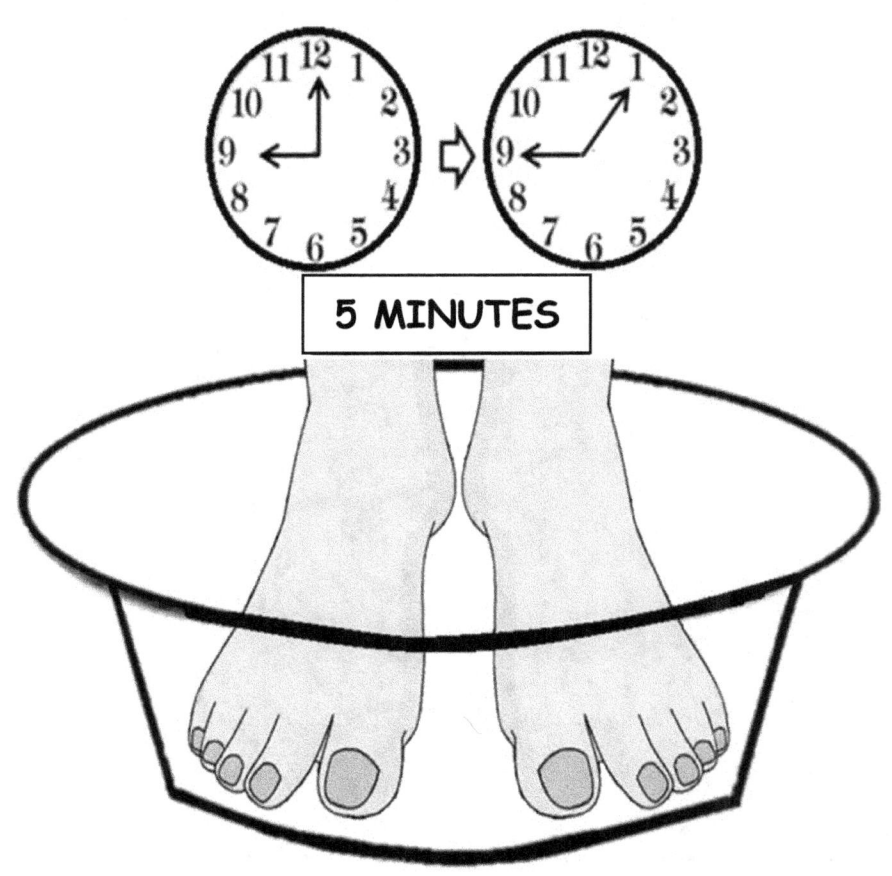

5 MINUTES

ADVICE #2
WASH YOUR FEET DAILY FOR 5 MINUTES, SUBMERGING THEM IN A WASHBOWL CONTAINING WARM SOAPY WATER, PUTTING SPECIAL EMPHASIS BETWEEN THE TOES.

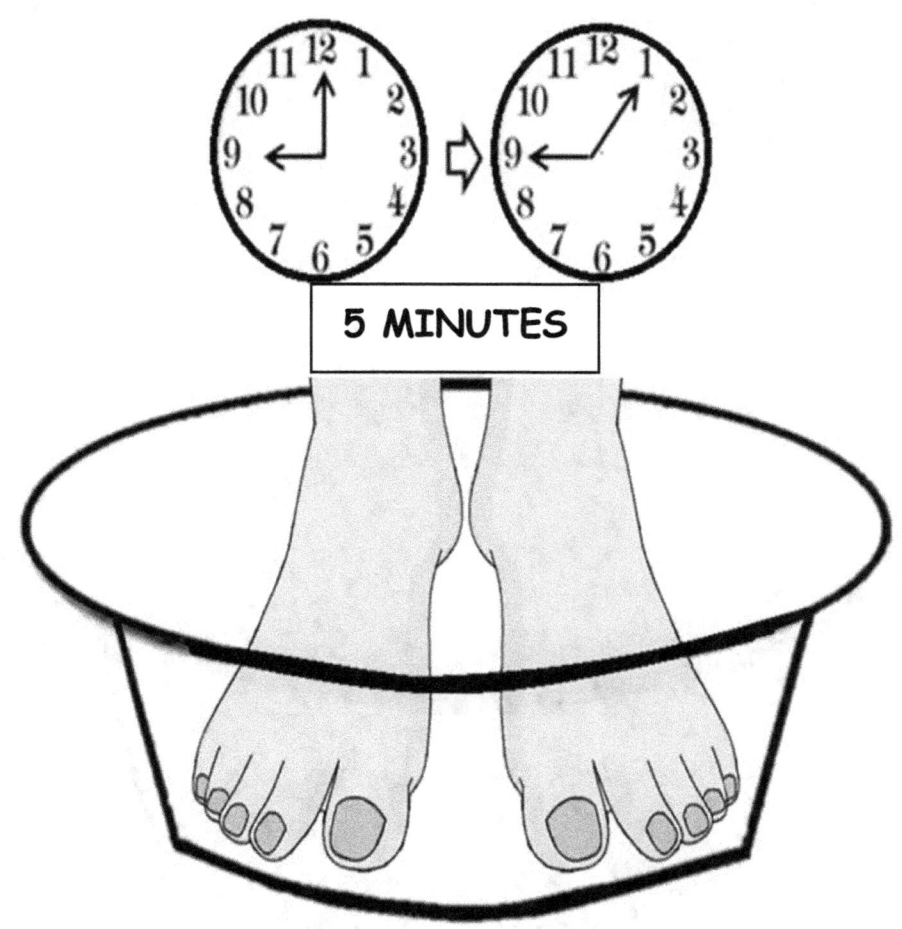

5 MINUTES

ADVICE #3
> AVOID THE USE OF SOAPS WITH HEAVY
INGREDIENTS.
> IF YOU HAVE VERY DRY SKIN USE A
MOISTURIZING SOAP (WHICH PRODUCES
HUMIDITY), IF YOUR PHYSICIAN OR
PODIATRIC RECOMMENDED.

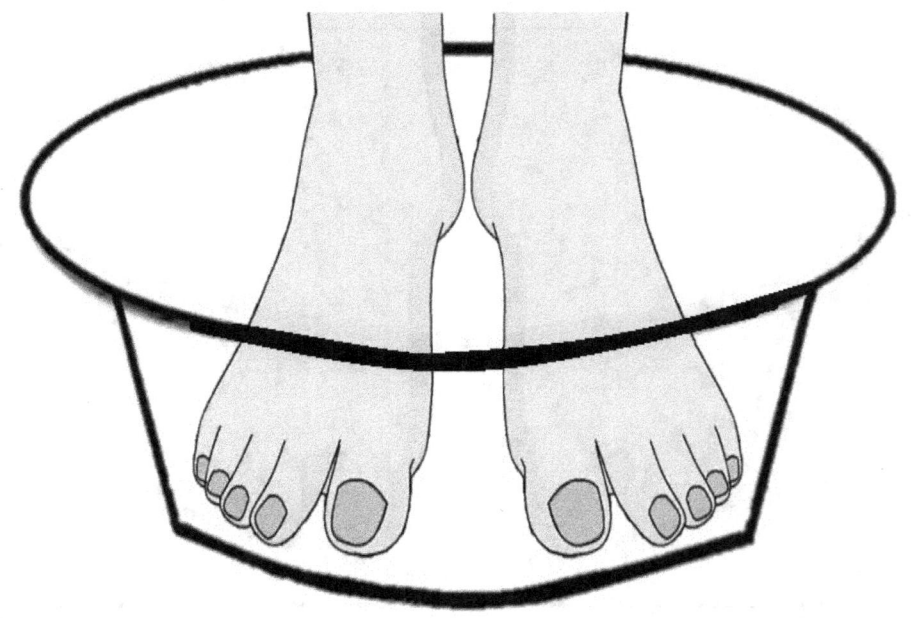

ADVICE #3. CONTINUATION.
IF NECESSARY, IN THIS HYGIENIC
ACTIVITY, UTILIZE THE HELP OF A FAMILY
MEMBER, NURSING ASSISTANT OF THE
HEALTH PLAN TO WHICH YOU BELONG OR
A FRIEND.

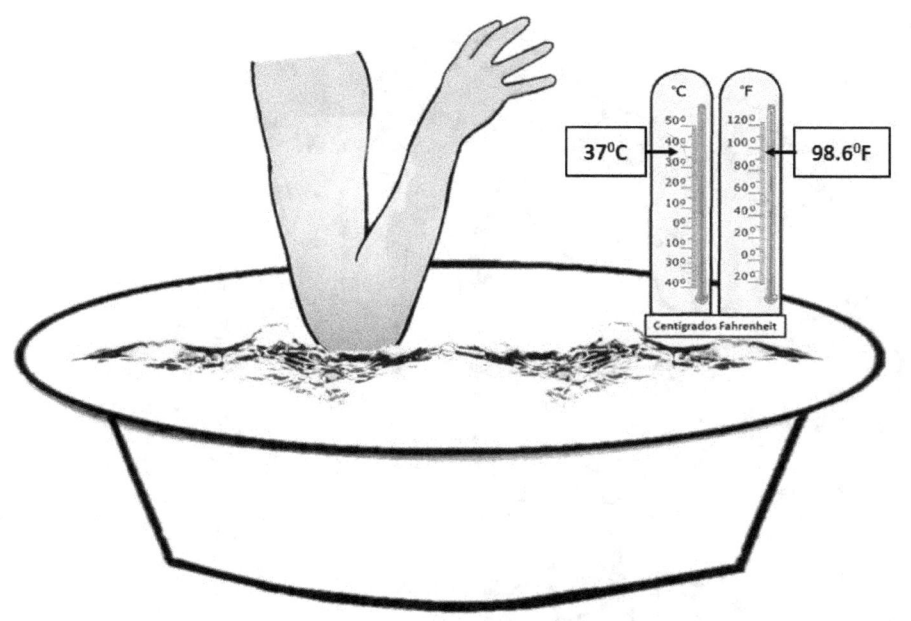

ADVICE #4
> BEFORE DIPPING YOUR FEET, CHECK THE WATER TEMPERATURE WITH A PART OF YOUR BODY OR WITH A THERMOMETER TO PREVENT BURNING YOUR SKIN.
> A TEMPERATURE NO MORE THAN 37 DEGREES CELSIUS OR 98.6 FAHRENHEIT, IS ADEQUATE.

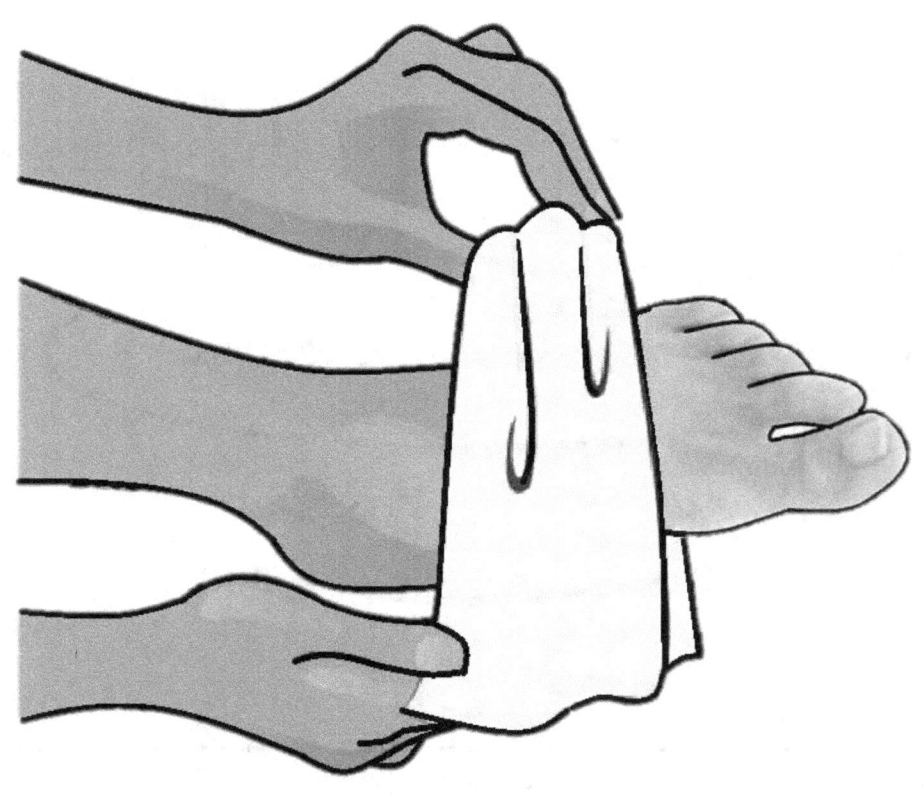

ADVICE #5
DRY YOUR FEET WELL WITH A SOFT
FABRIC TOWEL (COTTON), WITHOUT
FROTHING, APPLYING DISCRETE PRESSURE
OR GIVING PATHS TO ABSORB WATER AND
PLACE SPECIAL EMPHASIS ON THE AREA
BETWEEN THE TOES.

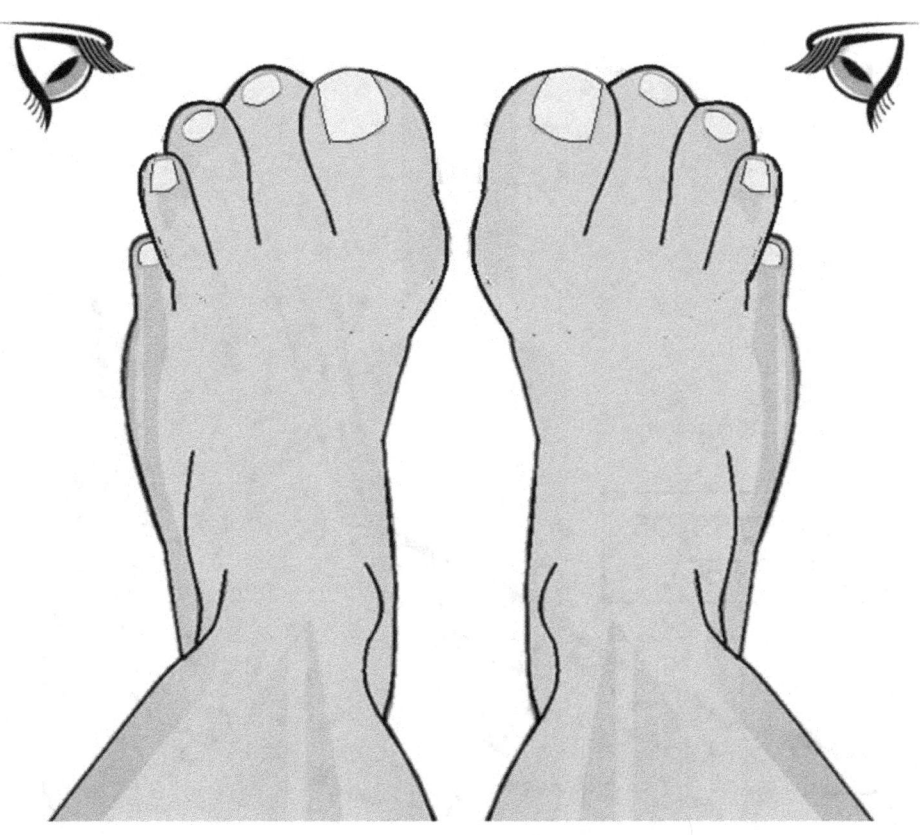

ADVICE #6

> CHECK YOUR FEET EVERY DAY, AFTER WASHING THEM.

> IF YOU HAVE DIFFICULTY LEANING OR LIFTING THE FEET TO OBSERVE THEM FOR SUFFER FROM ARTHRITIS, ARTHROSIS, OBESITY, OR IF THE DIABETES HAS AFFECTED YOUR VISION, REQUEST A FAMILY MEMBER'S HELP IN THE HOUSE OR REQUEST THE ATTENTION OF A NURSING ASSISTANT TO YOUR HEALTH PLAN.

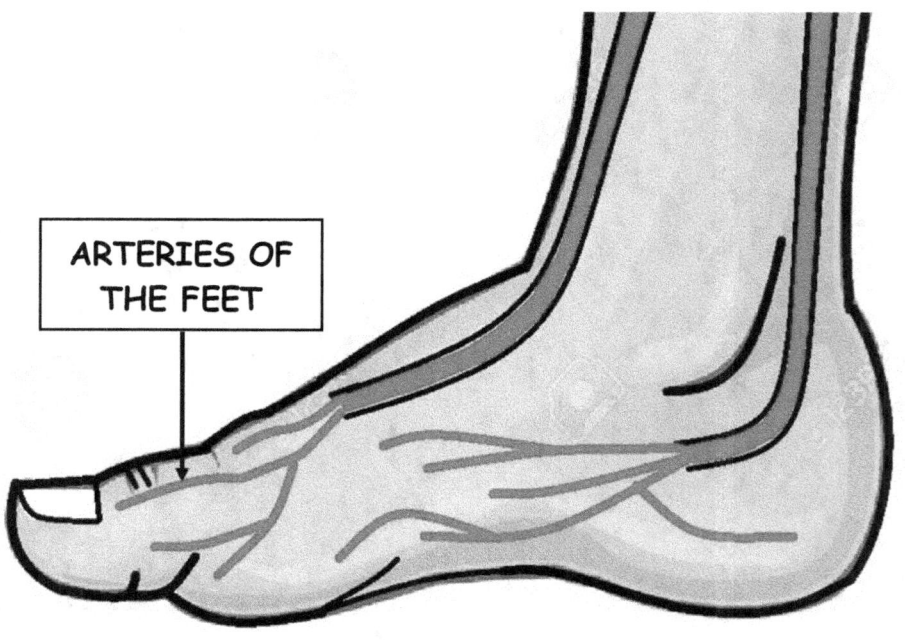

ARTERIES OF
THE FEET

ADVICE #7
> WHEN YOU GO TO YOUR DOCTOR'S
APPOINTMENT, ASK THE DOCTOR IF YOU
HAVE PROBLEMS WITH THE ARTERIAL
CIRCULATION IN YOUR FEET (PERIPHERAL
ARTERIAL DISEASE).
> KNOWING THIS WILL FACILITATE THE
INSPECTION AND INTERPRETATION OF
THE FINDINGS RELATED TO THIS
CONDITION.

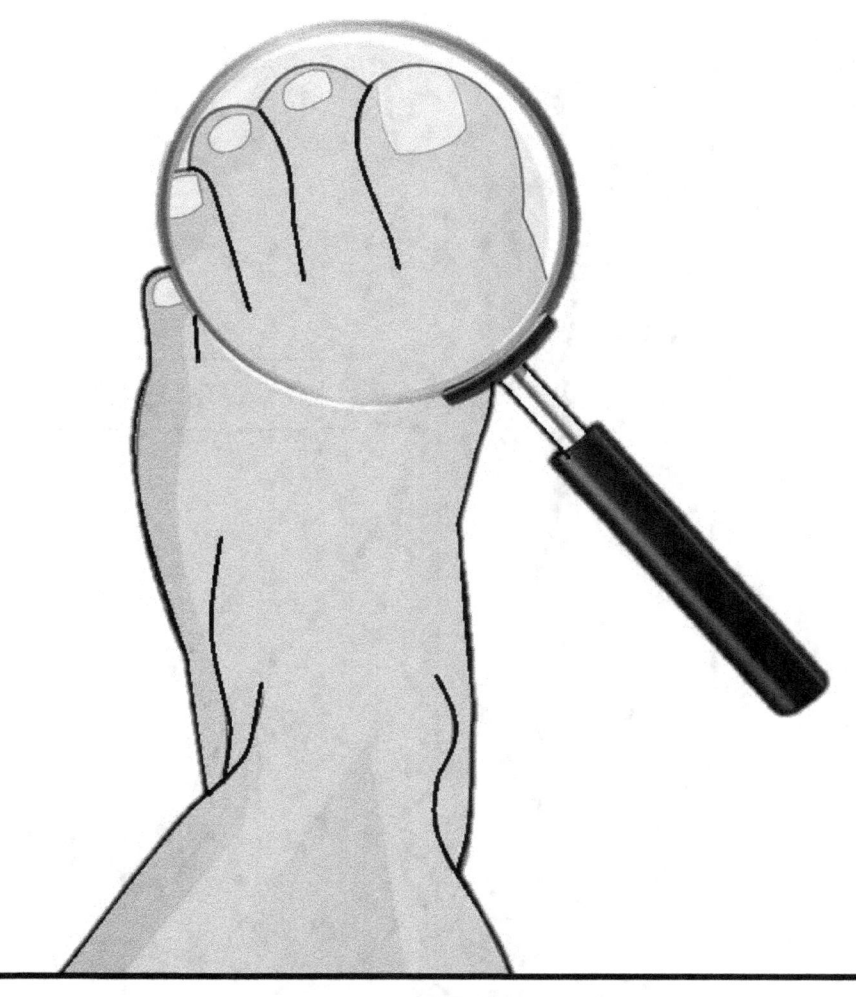

ADVICE #8
> LOOKING AT THE FOOT, INVESTIGATE:
> THE COLOR OF YOUR SKIN: IF IT IS RED, BLUE, PALE (WHITE).
> THE TEXTURE OF YOUR SKIN (SENSATION THAT PRODUCE THE TOUCH): IF THE SKIN IS RUGGED, VERY DRY, COLD OR HOT.

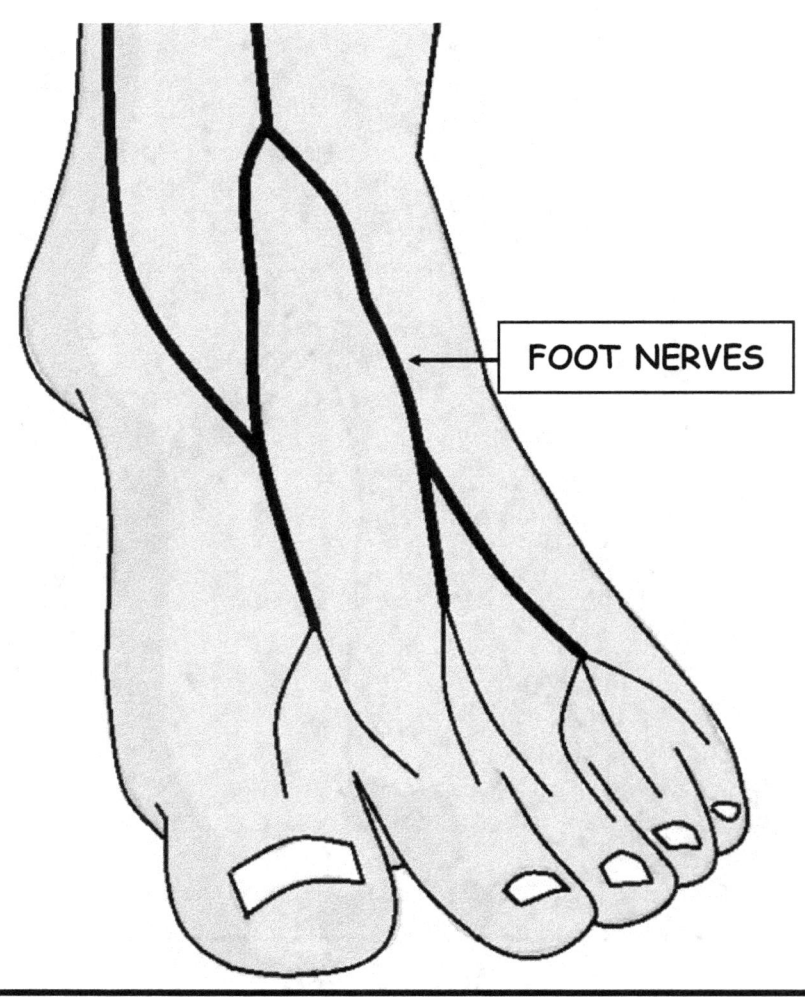

FOOT NERVES

ADVICE #9
> WHEN YOU HAVE AN APPOINTMENT WITH YOUR PHYSICIAN, ASK IF YOU HAVE DAMAGE TO THE NERVES OF YOUR FEET (DIABETIC NEUROPATHY).
TO INSPECT YOUR FEET PROPERLY, YOU NEED TO KNOW IT.

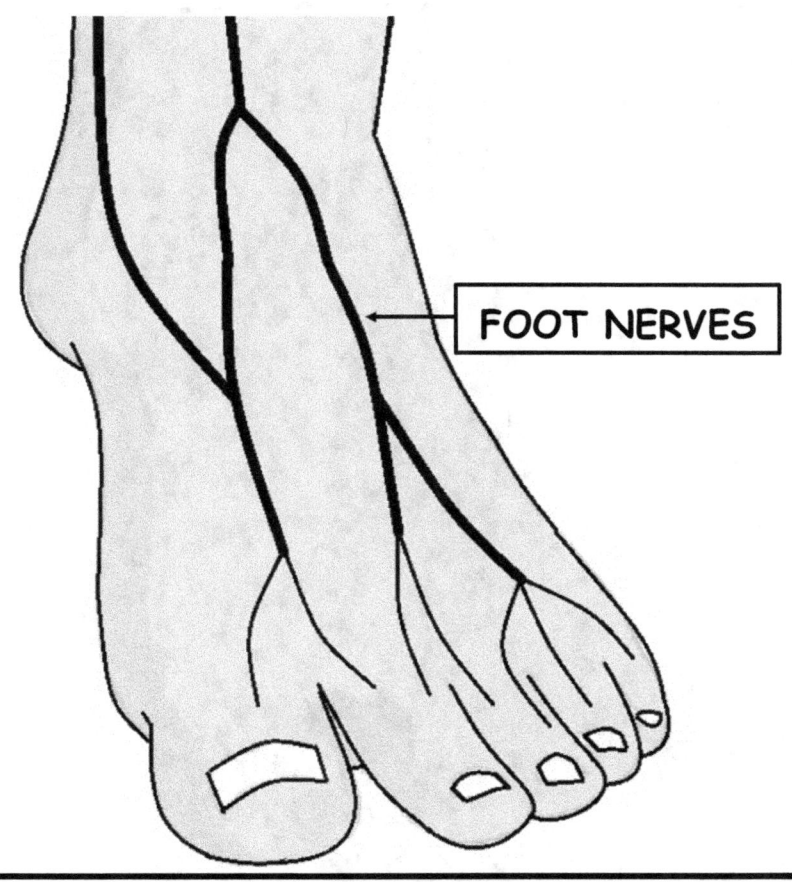

FOOT NERVES

ADVICE #9. CONTINUATION.
IF YOU HAVE DAMAGE TO YOUR NERVES
YOU WILL LOSE SENSITIVITY:
TACTILE, IF WHEN YOU TOUCH YOUR
FOOT, YOU DO NOT FEEL THE CONTACT.
PAINFUL, TIGHTEN AND DOES NOT
PERCEIVE PAIN (ANESTHESIA)
AND THERMAL, IT IS FLAMMABLE AND
DOES NOT APPRECIATE THE TEMPERATURE
INCREASE.

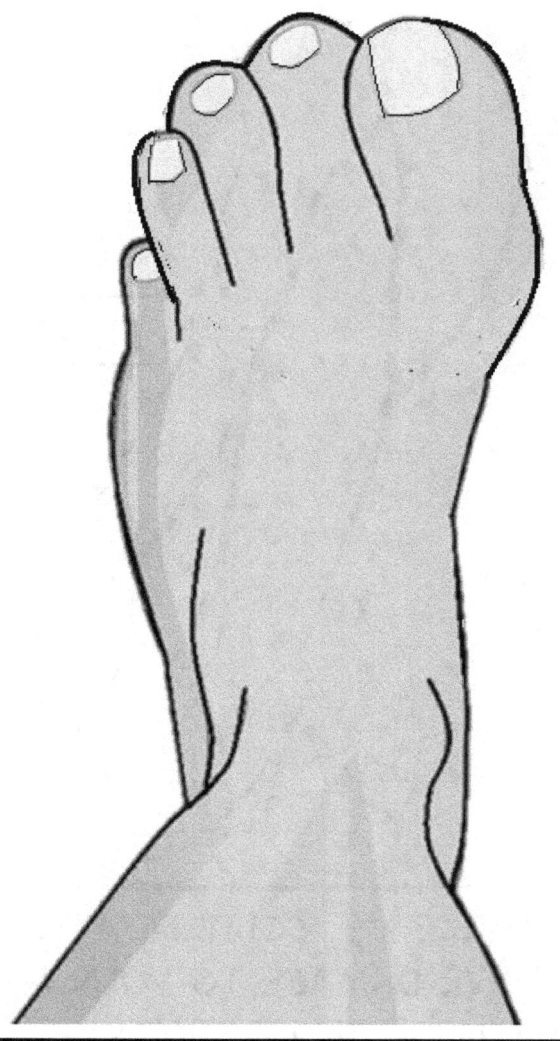

ADVICE #10

> WATCH OUT:

> IF THERE IS LOSS OF THE HAIR IN TOES, FOOT OR LOWER THIRD OF THE LEG.

> IF THERE IS ANY CHANGE IN THE SHAPE OR THE SIZE OF YOUR FOOT.

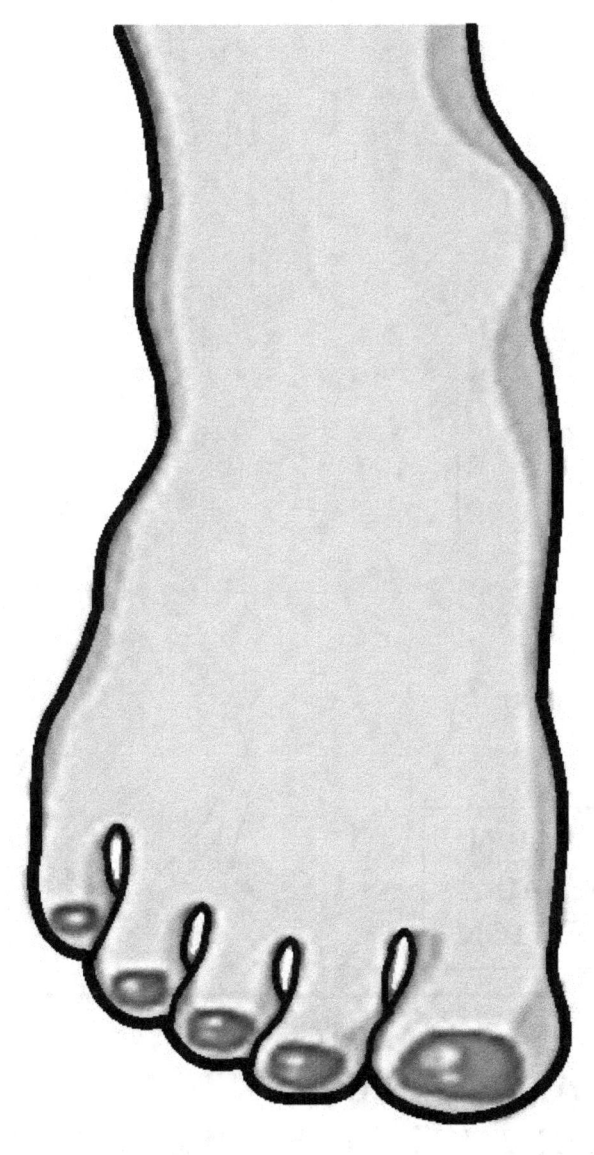

ADVICE #11
DO NOT PAINT THE FOOT'S NAILS, THIS
COULD HIDE IMPORTANT ALTERATIONS
AND MAKE IT HARD TO INSPECT THEM.

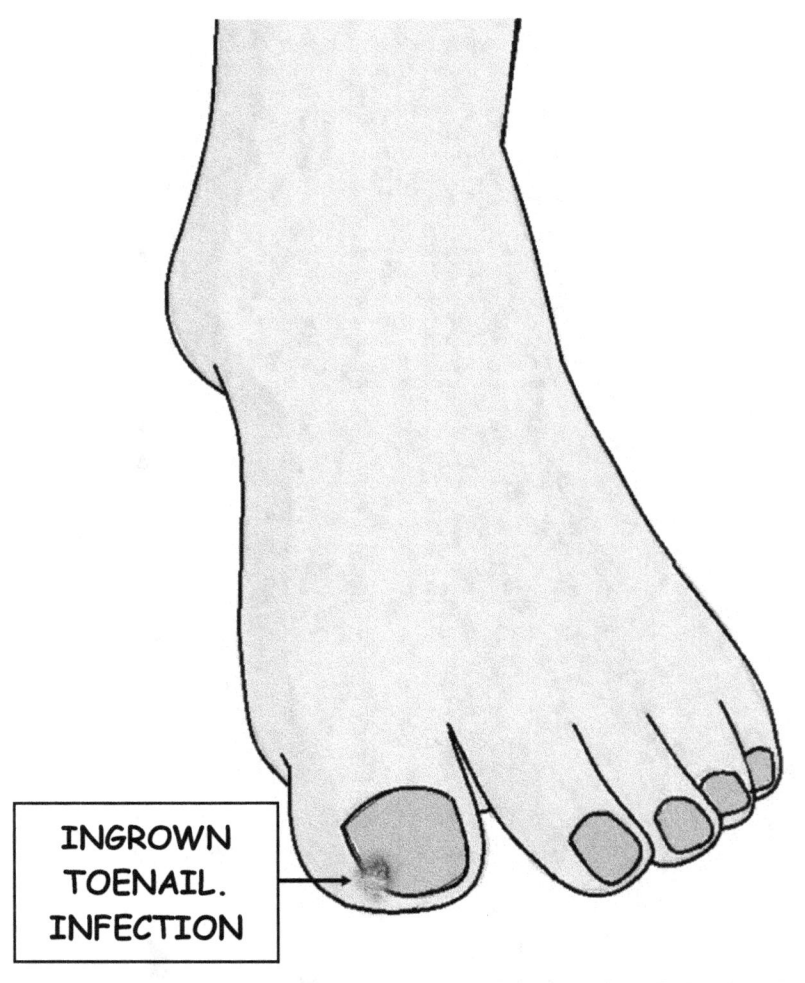

INGROWN TOENAIL. INFECTION

ADVICE #12
> LOOK AT YOUR FEET, SEE IF:
>THE NAILS ARE GROSS, WITH CHANGES OR COLORATION OR BURSTED IN THE BORDERS WITH INFLAMMATION SIGNS.
> IF YOU DETECT SOME OF THESE SYMPTOMS, CONSULT WITH YOUR PRIMARY PHYSICIAN OR WITH A PODIATRIST.

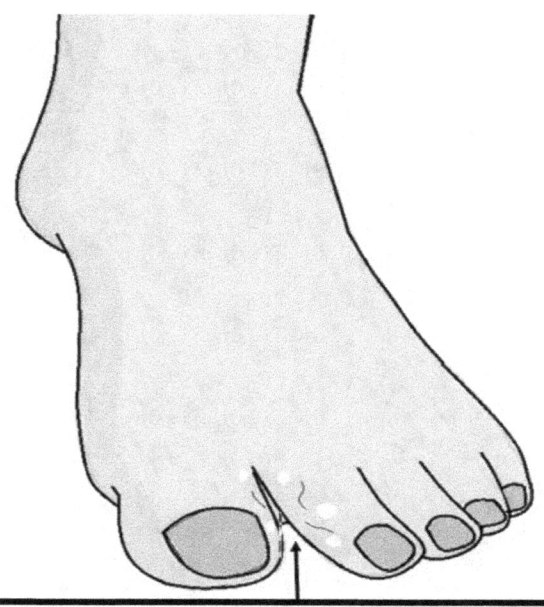

FUNGI. CRACKERS AND DECAMATION

ADVICE #13

> WHEN CONTEMPLATING THE FEET, WATCH OUT:

> IF THERE ARE SYMPTOMS THAT MAKE YOU THINK THAT THERE IS A FUNGUS IN THE NAILS OR BETWEEN THE TOES, SUCH AS: ITCH, EXCESSIVE HUMIDITY, MACERATION OF SKIN (SOFT SKIN AND HUMIDITY), FLAKES OR CRUST, OR RIVEN (CRACKS) AND BLISTERS WITHOUT OR WITH OUTLET OF LIQUIDS.

> IF YOU DETECT SOME OF THESE SYMPTOMS, CONSULT WITH YOUR PRIMARY PHYSICIAN OR WITH A PODIATRIST.

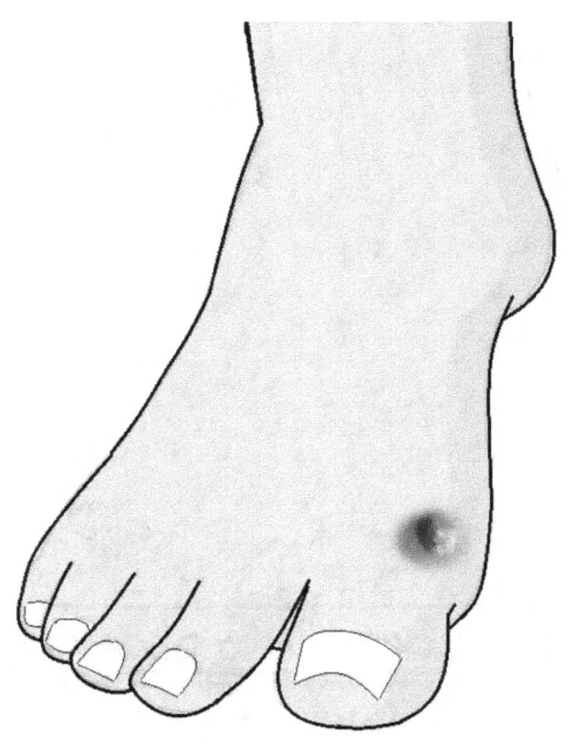

ADVICE #14

-OBSERVE IF THERE IS SOME SITE ON THE SKIN OF THE FOOT WITH SIGNS OF INFECTION:

> <u>LOCAL SIGNS</u>: INCREASE IN VOLUME, IN TEMPERATURE, REDNESS, PALPATION PAIN, SKIN OPENING, SUPURATION, OR BAD ODOR.

> <u>GENERAL SYMPTOMS</u>: DECOMPENSATION OF DIABETES, FEVER, SHIVERS, PHYSICAL DISCOMFORT, LACK OF ENERGY, LACK OF APPETITE.

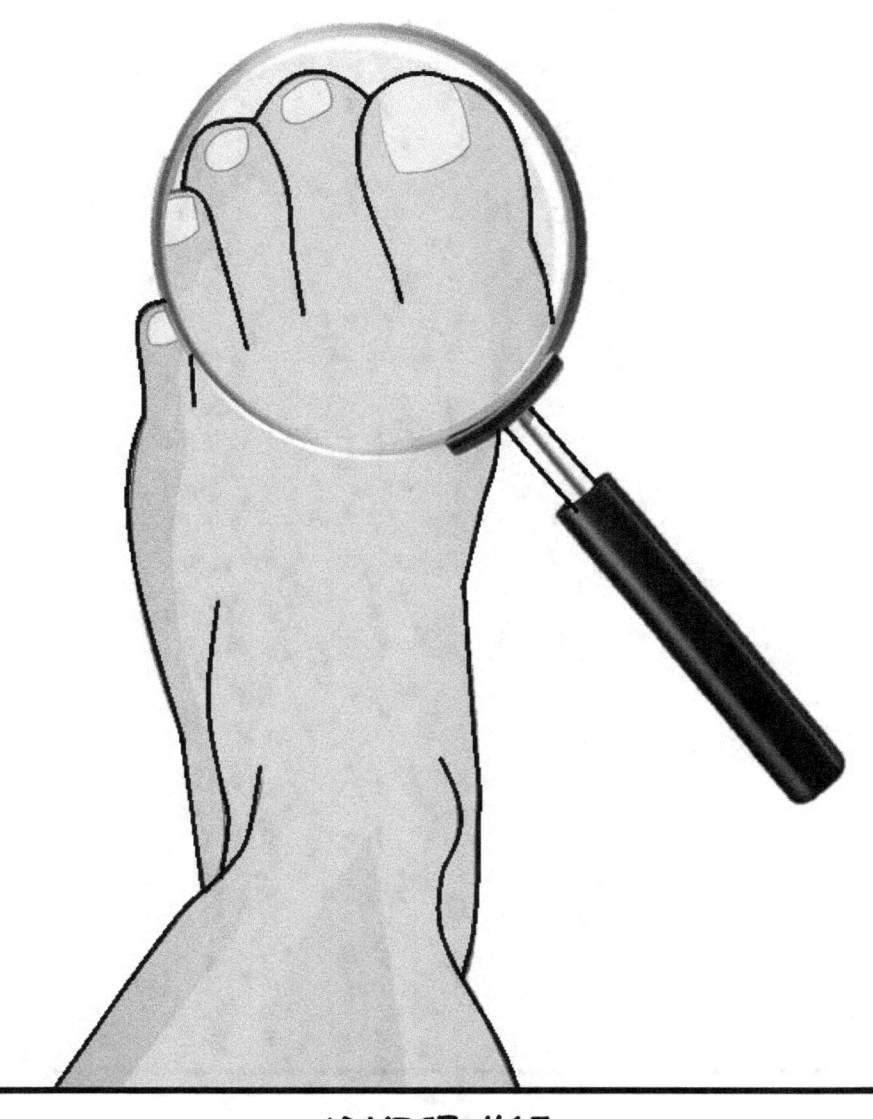

ADVICE #15
LOOK FOR THE PRESENCE OF ANY
INJURIES:
IRRITATED ZONES, BLISTERS, TOUCH OR
PRESSURE SITES, ULCERS, CRACKS,
CALLOSITY OR CALLUS.

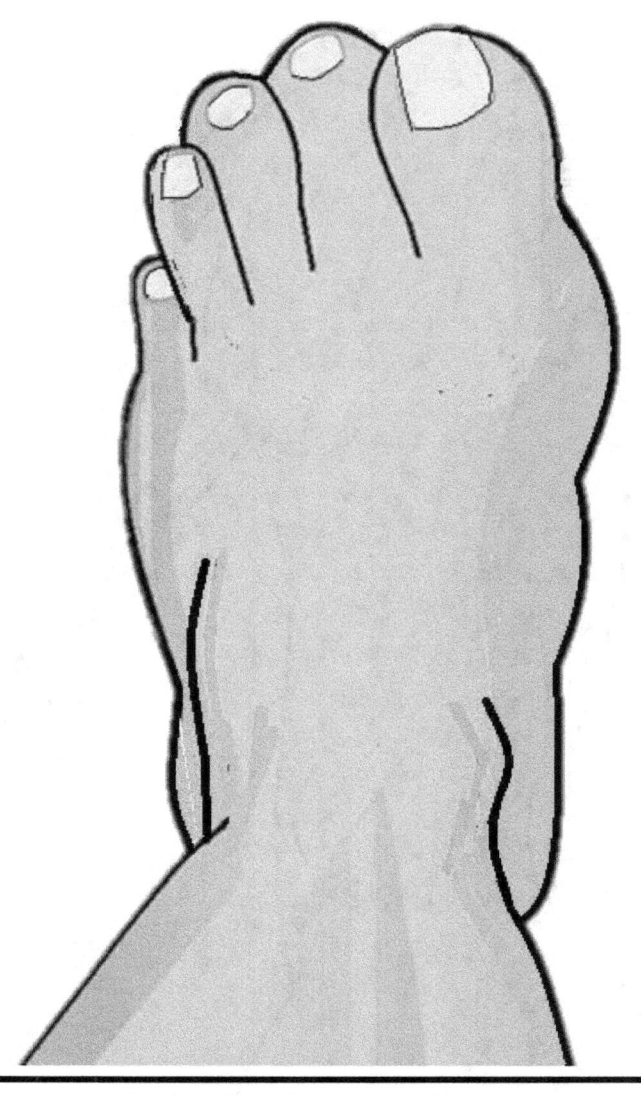

ADVICE #16
OBSERVE IF THE FOOT IS SWOLLEN
(EDEMA ON A FOOT ONLY), AND IF YOU
APPLY A DISCRETE PRESSURE WITH YOUR
INDEX FINGER IN THE ANKLE, IF IT
MAKES A DEPRESSION OR A LITTLE HOLE.

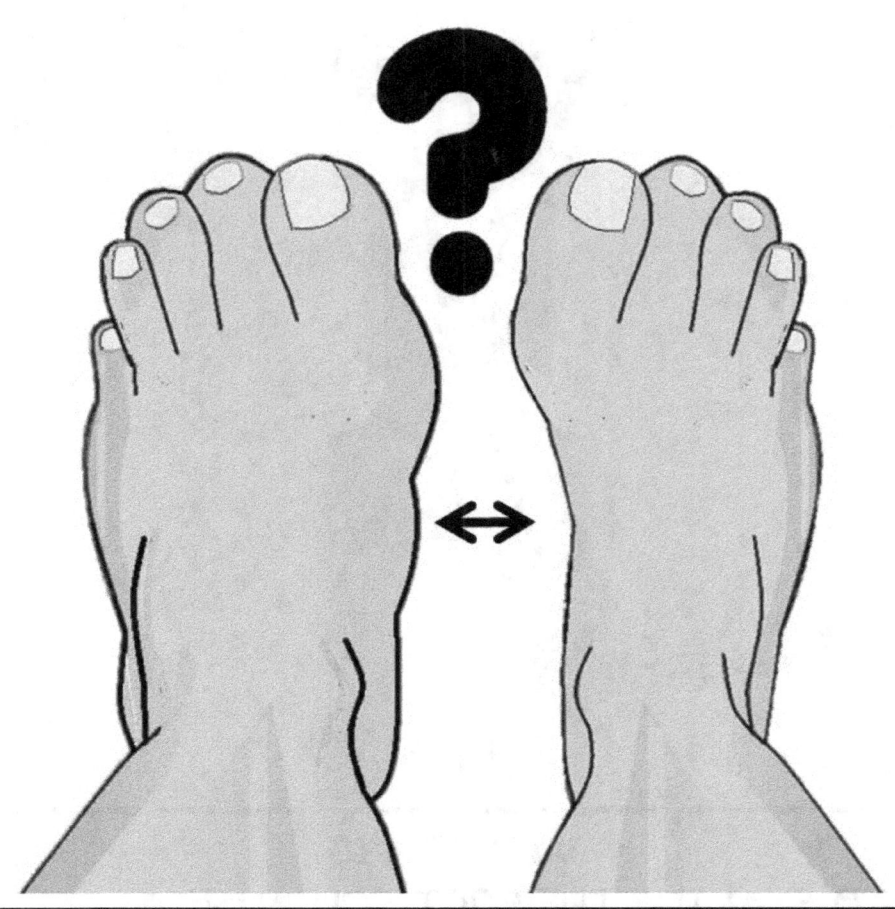

ADVICE #17
IF YOU HAVE DOUBTS ABOUT SOME
FINDINGS, COMPARE ONE FOOT WITH THE
OTHER, IF THE OTHER IS HEALTHY.

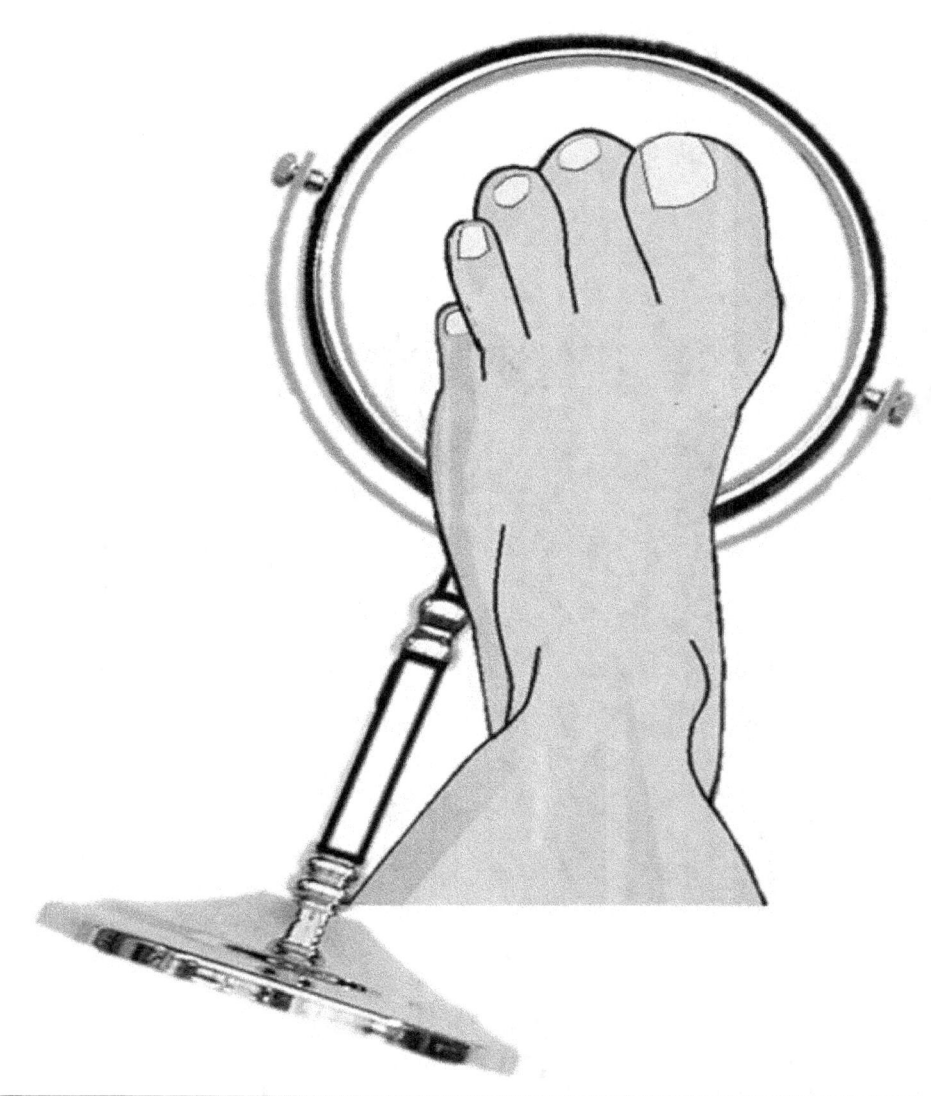

ADVICE #18
TO EXAMINE THE FOOT SOLE, USE A
LARGE MAGNIFYING MIRROR.
IF IT IS VERY HARD TO HOLD, PLACE IT
ON THE FLOOR TO FACILITATE THE
OBSERVATION.

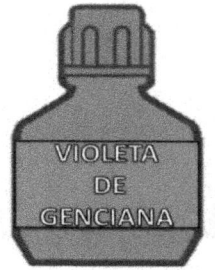
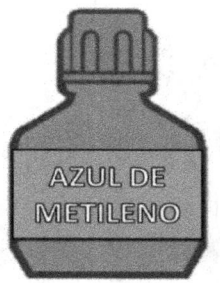
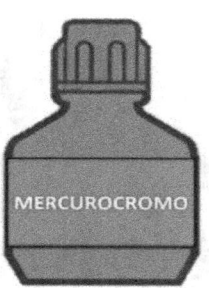

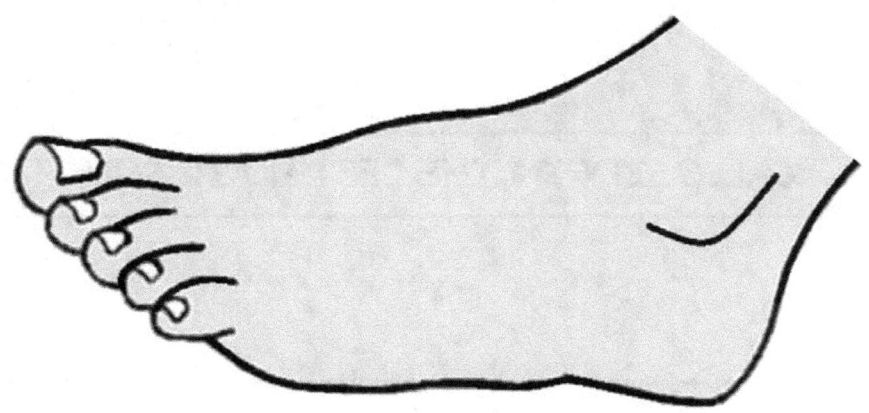

ADVICE #19
DO NOT APPLY ANY CREAM OR LOTION
THAT MODIFIES SKIN COLORING AND
DISGUISES OR CONFUSES WHEN
INSPECTING YOUR FEET.

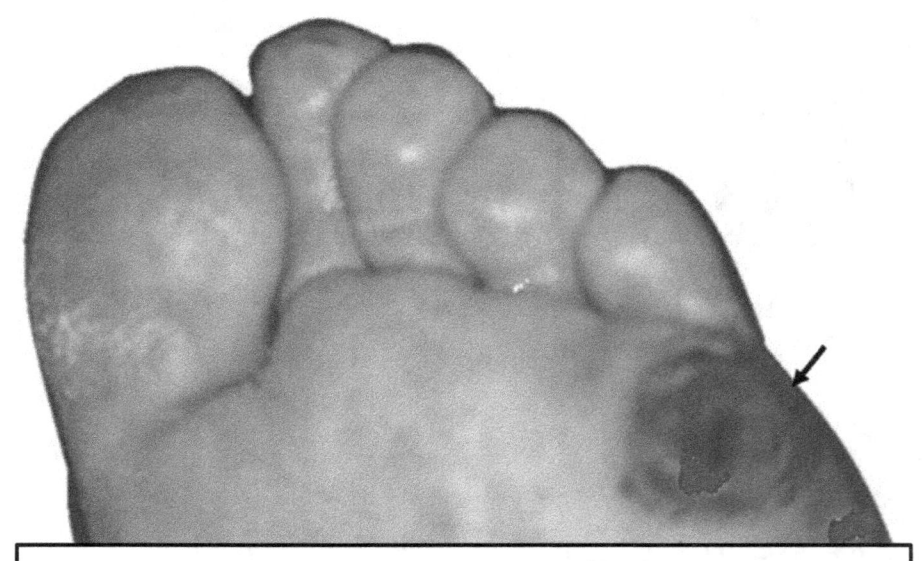

CALLOSITY IN THE LEFT FOOT SOLE

ADVICE #20
CONSULT YOUR PRIMARY PHYSICIAN OR
YOUR PODIATRIST ABOUT ANY CALLOSITY
OR CALLUS AT YOUR FEET. IF THESE
APPEAR, IT IS INDICATIVE THAT IN THAT
ZONE THERE EXISTS A PRESSURE OR
GRAZE INADEQUATE.

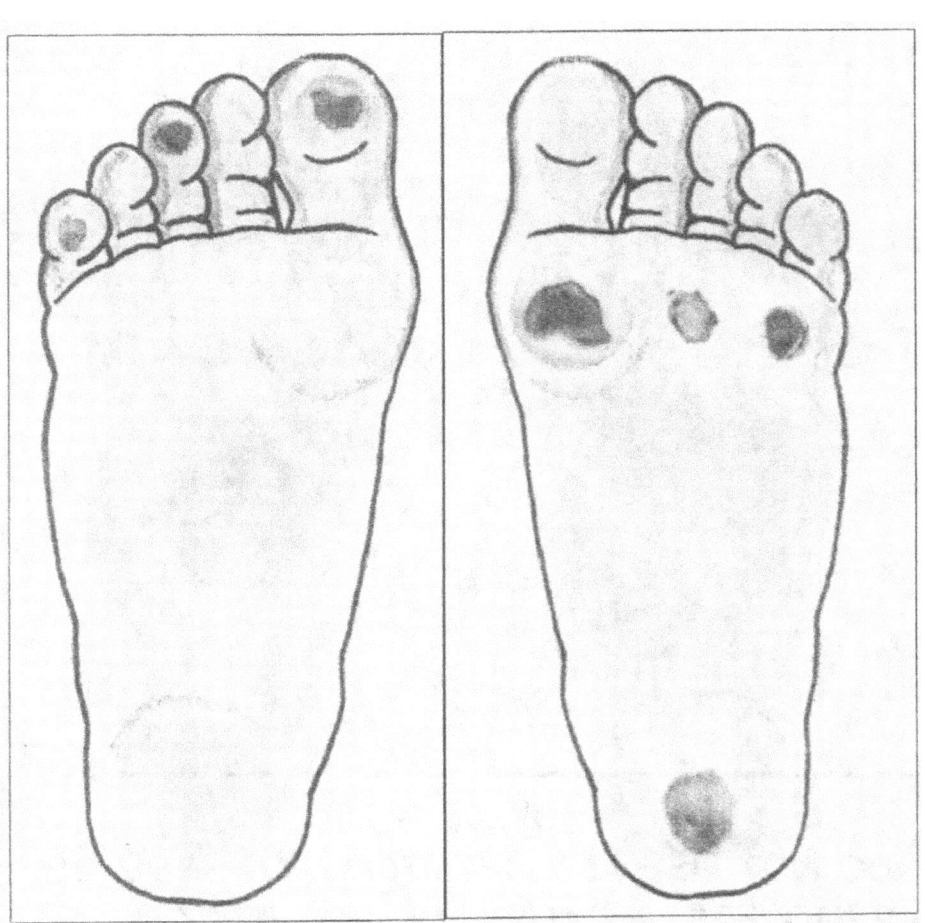

THE MOST COMMON LOCATIONS OF
CALLOSITES AND PLANTAR ULCERS.

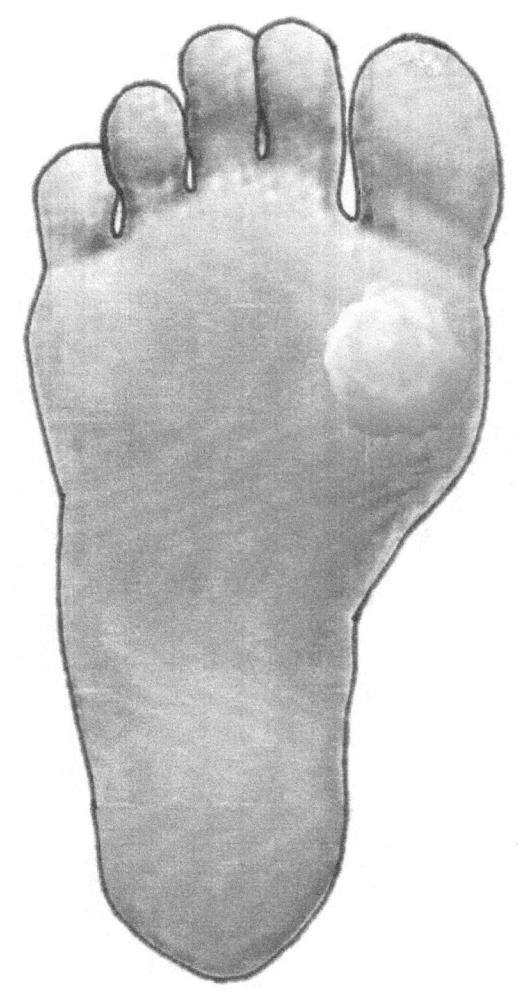

ADVICE # 21
DO NOT USE ANY CHEMICALS OR LIQUIDS,
REMOVERS, PATCHES, OR MECHANICAL
METHODS TO REDUCE CALLOSITES OR
CALLUS WITHOUT CONSULTING YOUR
DOCTOR OR PODIATRIST, DUE TO THE
POSSIBILITY OF CAUSING AN INJURY.

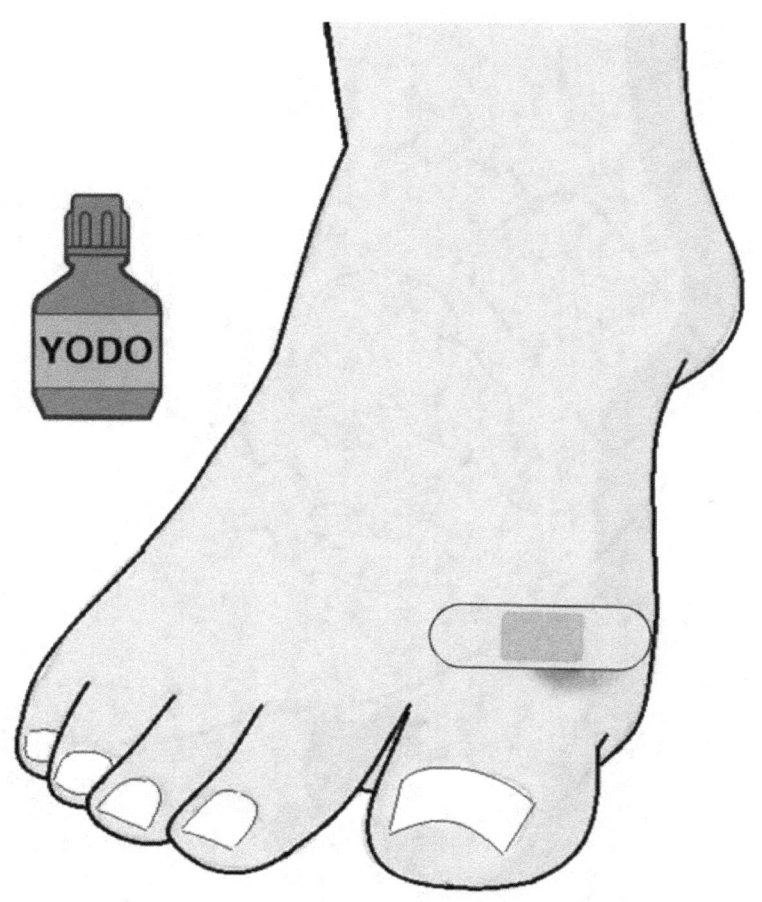

ADVICE #22

>AVOID THE USE OF STRONG OR IRRITANT ANTISEPTICS IN FOOT INJURIES WITHOUT CONSULTING WITH YOUR PHYSICIAN OR PODIATRISTT.
> DO NOT APPLY ADHESIVE BANDAGES OR ADHESIVE TAPE IN FOOT INFECTIONS, WHICH COULD CAUSE AN INJURY TO THE ADJACENT SKIN.

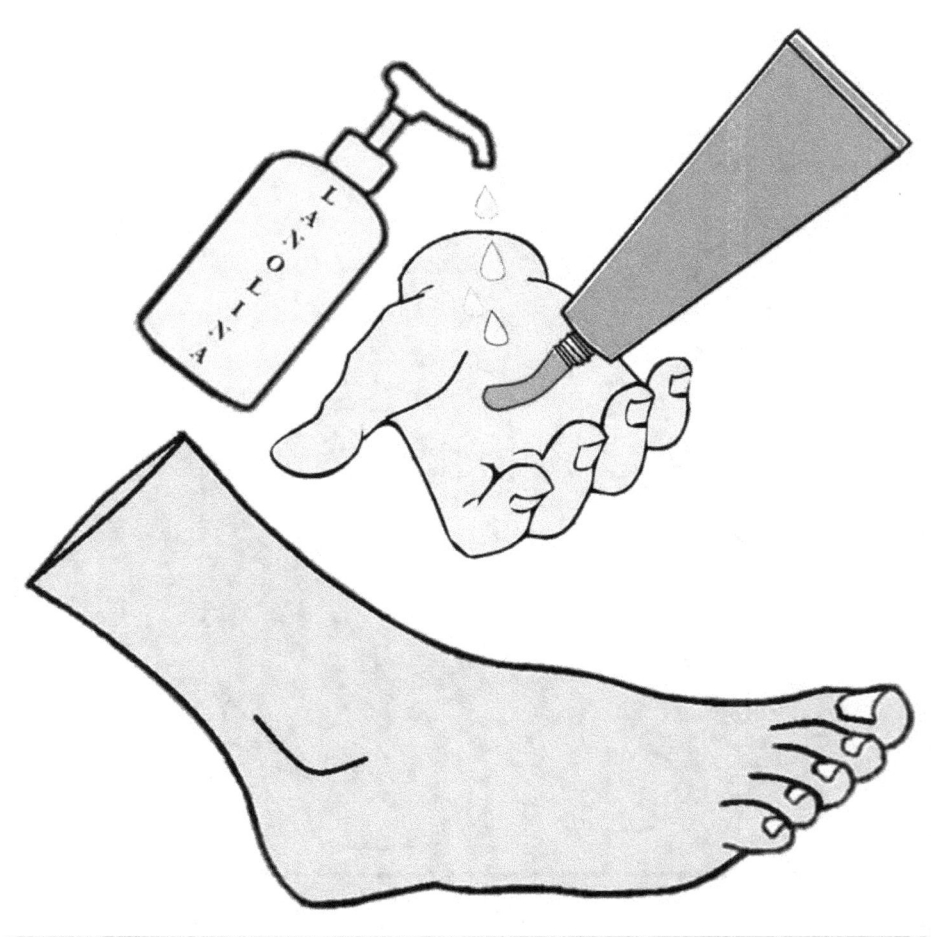

ADVICE #23

AFTER EXAMINING YOUR FEET, GIVE SOFT MASSAGES WITH A LOTION, CREAM OR PRESCRIPTINO ORDER RECOMMENDED BY YOUR PHYSICIAN OR THE PODIATRIST, ESPECIALLY WHERE THERE IS CALLOSITIES, DRYING AND CRACKS. DO NOT APPLY BETWEEN THE TOES.

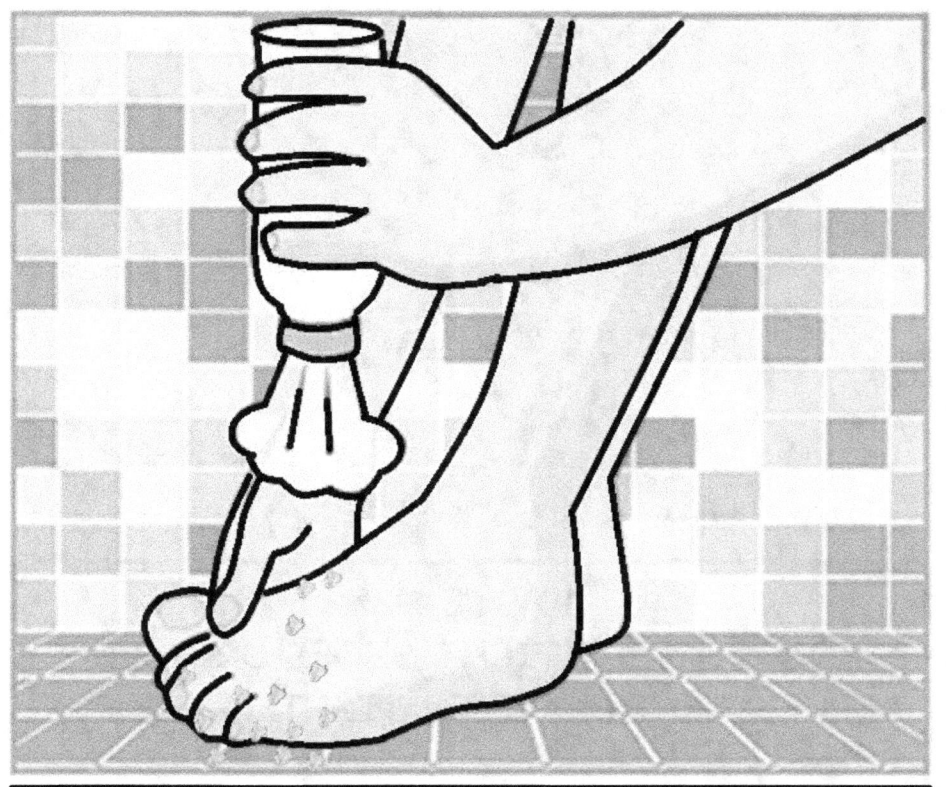

ADVICE #24.
ONCE THE DAILY MASSAGE IS FINISHED,
APPLY TALCUM POWDER ON THE FOOT,
BETWEEN THE TOES AND IF YOU PERSPIRE
TOO MUCH, DO IT TWO OR THREE TIMES
A DAY.

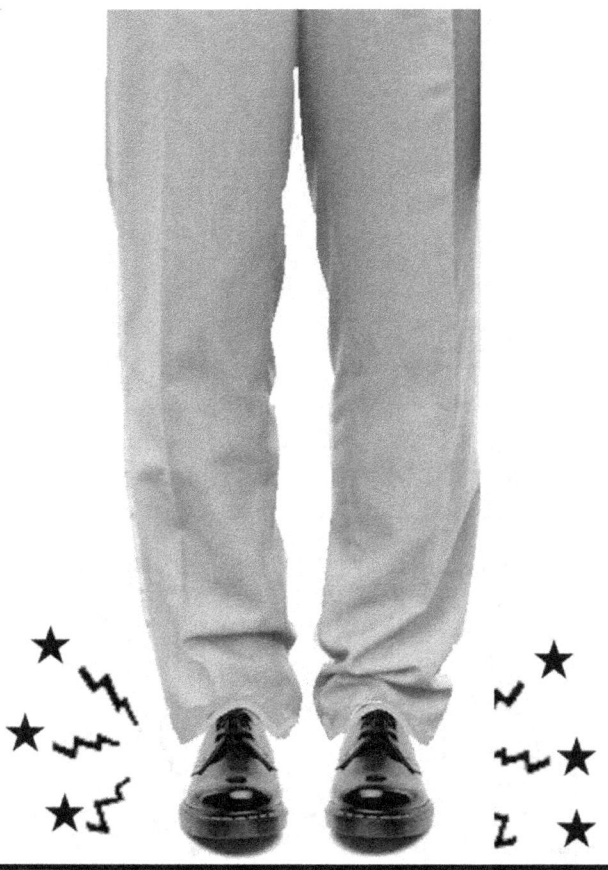

ADVICE #25

> DO NOT WEAR TIGHT SHOES OR HAVE STRAPS THAT GRAZE OR TIGHTEN THE SKIN.

> AVOID PUTTING SHOES WITHOUT USING SOCKS, IT MAY CAUSE BLISTERS OR INJURIES TO THE FEET.

> DO NOT USE LOOSE-FITTING SHOES THAT SWAY ON THE FOOT WHEN YOU WALK.

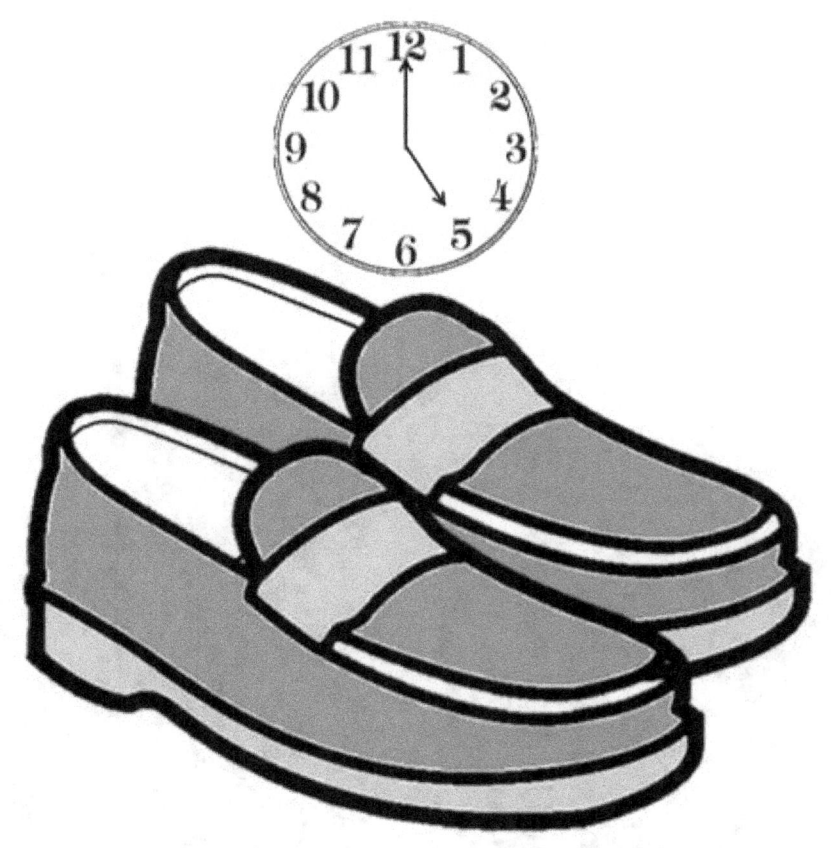

ADVICE #26

> BUY SHOES IN THE AFTERNOON HOURS, WHEN YOUR FEET ARE MORE SWOLLEN.

> ASK FOR A WIDE POINT AND SOFT SKIN SHOES, WITH LACES OR VELCRO TO BE ABLE TO ADJUST IT TO YOUR TASTE.

> IF YOU WEAR SUPPORTS, TAKE THEM TO THE STORE AND TRY ON THE SHOES WITH THEM INSIDE.

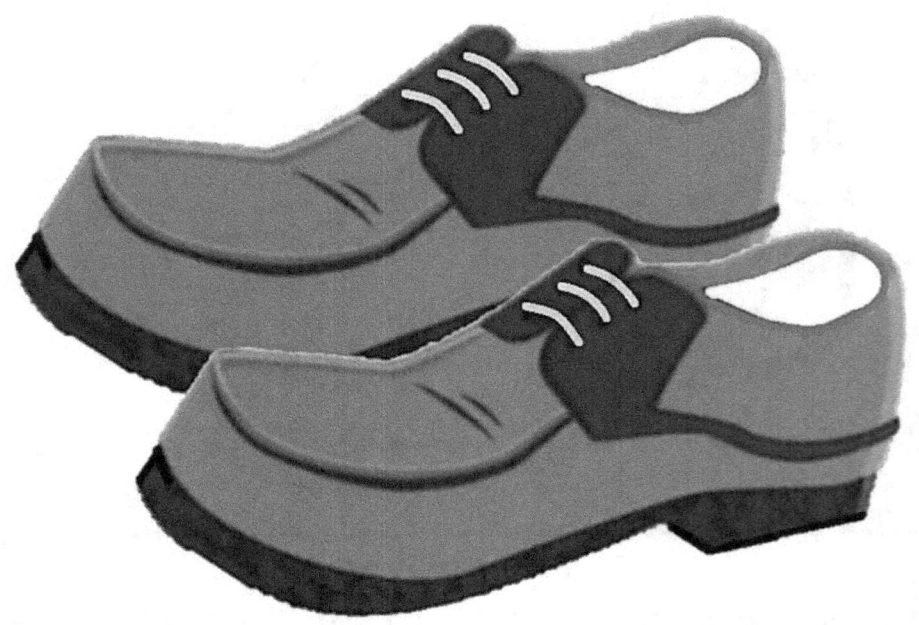

ADVICE #27
DURING THE PURCHASE OF SHOES
CONSIDER THE FOLLOWING
REQUIREMENTS:
THAT THE MATERIAL TRANSPIRES HEAT,
LOW HEELS (MAXIMUM 5 CM) AND
TEMPLATE PADDED.

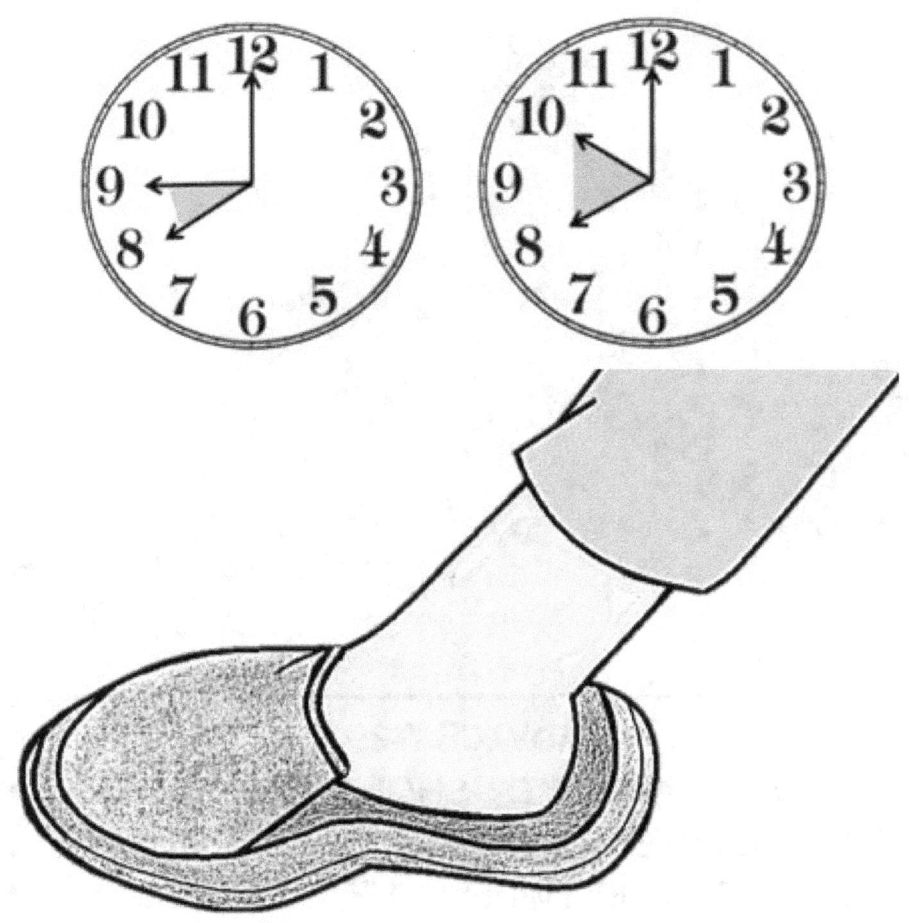

ADVICE #28
USE NEW SHOES ONLY 1 TO 2 HOURS THE
FIRST DAYS AND INCREASE HALF HOURS
EVERY THREE DAYS, IF THEY HAVE NOT
CAUSED ANY PROBLEMS.

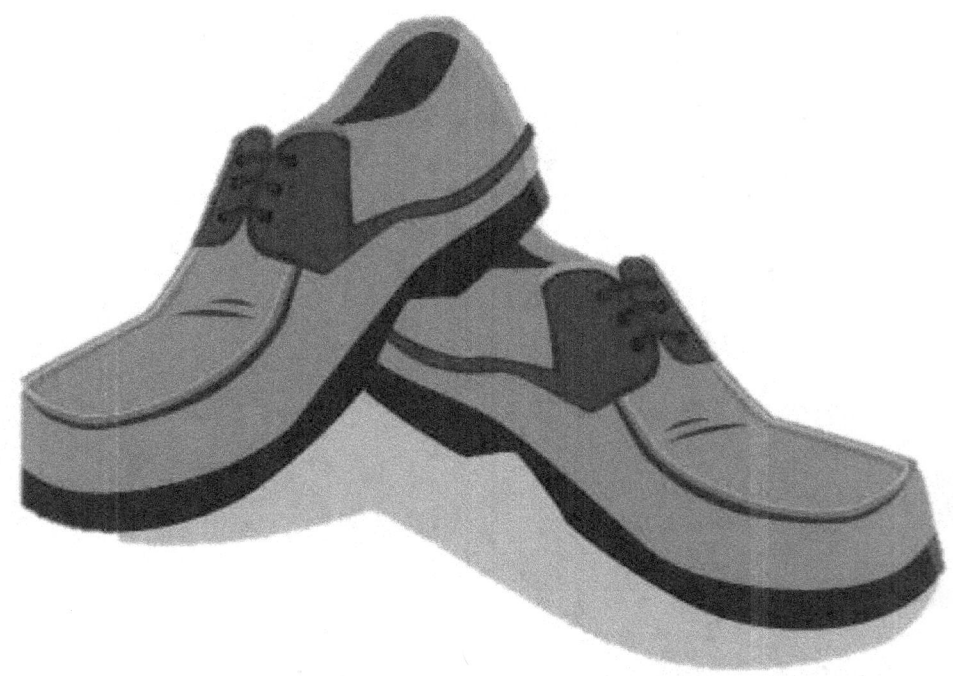

ADVICE #29

> AVOID HARD SKIN SHOES (PLASTICS), FINE POINTED, AS WELL AS SANDALS WITH BELTS BETWEEN THE FINGERS.

> SOFT LEATHER SHOES, TENNIS OR SPORTS SHOES ARE APPROPRIATE FOR USE.

> THE SHOES WITH ELASTIC CLOSURE MAKE IT EASY TO PUT THEM ON AND REMOVE THEM.

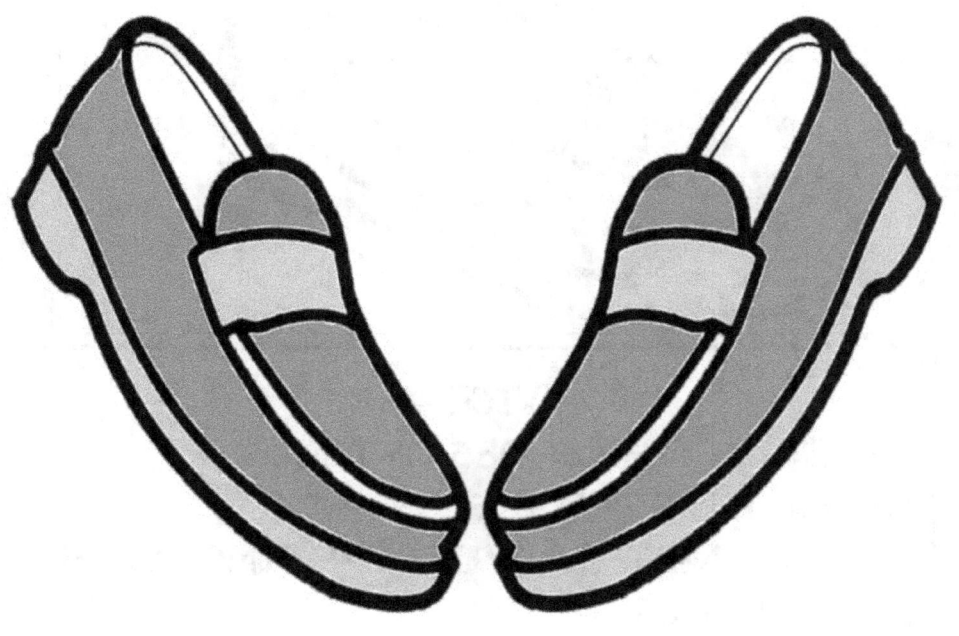

ADVICE #30
CHANGE SHOES TWICE A DAY TO SWITCH
THE SUPPORT POINTS AND SCRAPES WITH
A SAME TYPE OF SHOE.

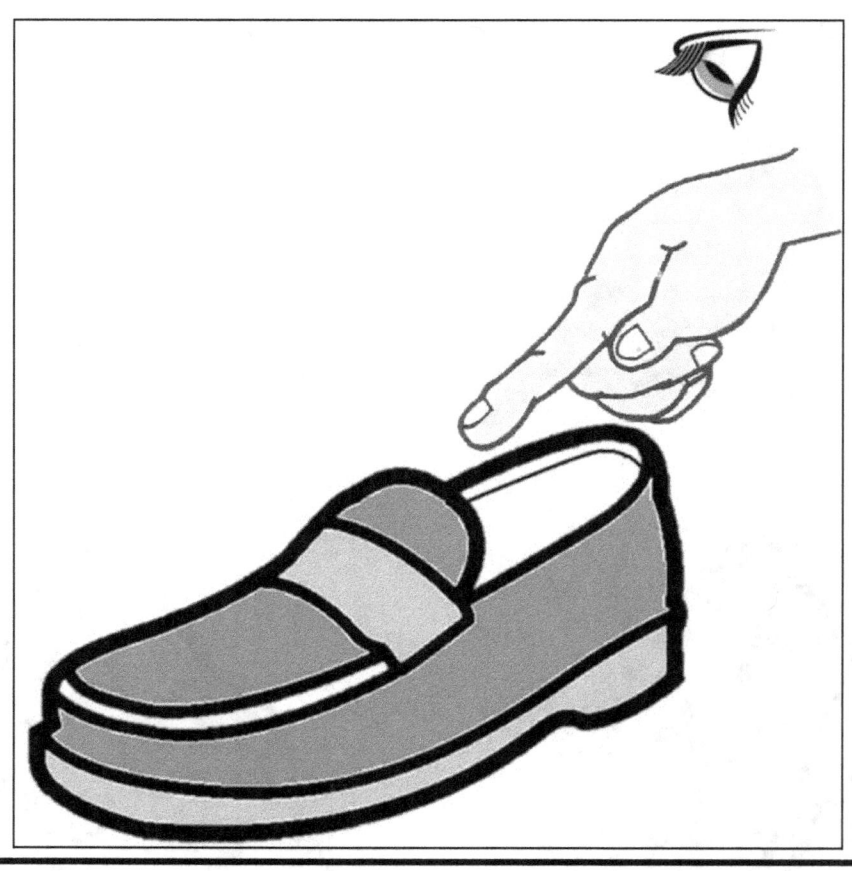

ADVICE #31
NEVER USE THE SHOES WITHOUT
OBSERVING THEM INSIDE AND
INSPECTING THEM WITH THE FINGERS IN
ITS INTERIOR.
INVESTIGATE THE PRESENCE OF ANY
SHARP OBJECT, LITTLE STONE, WRINKLES
IN THE INTERNAL SOLE OR PRONOUNCED
EDGE THAT MAY CAUSE INJURY.

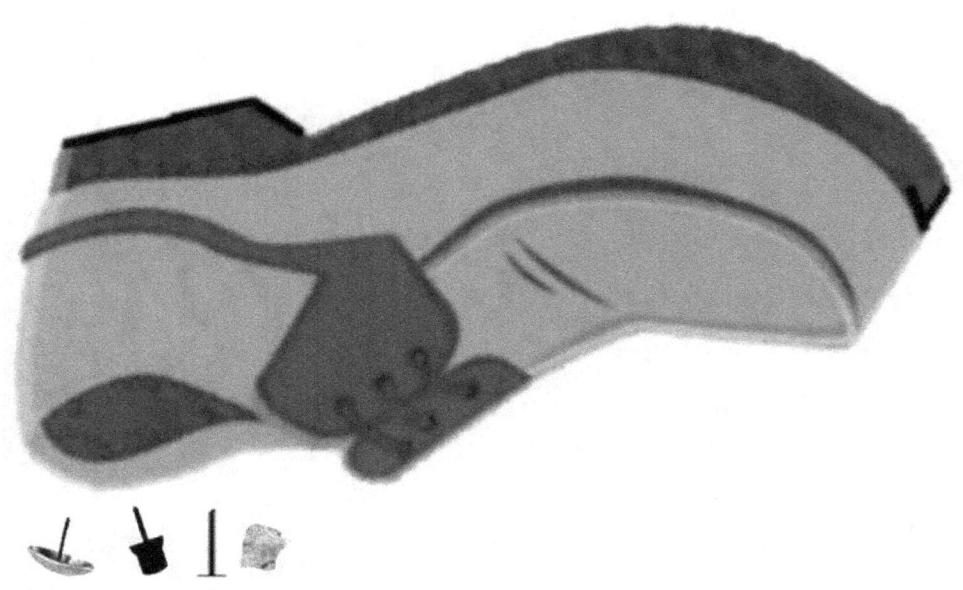

ADVISE #32
PLACE THE SHOES INTO THE INVERTED
POSITION AND SHAKE THEM SEVERAL
TIMES TRYING TO EXPEL ANY FOREIGN
BODY THAT COULD BE INSIDE IT AND TO
CAUSE AN INJURY TO THE FOOT.

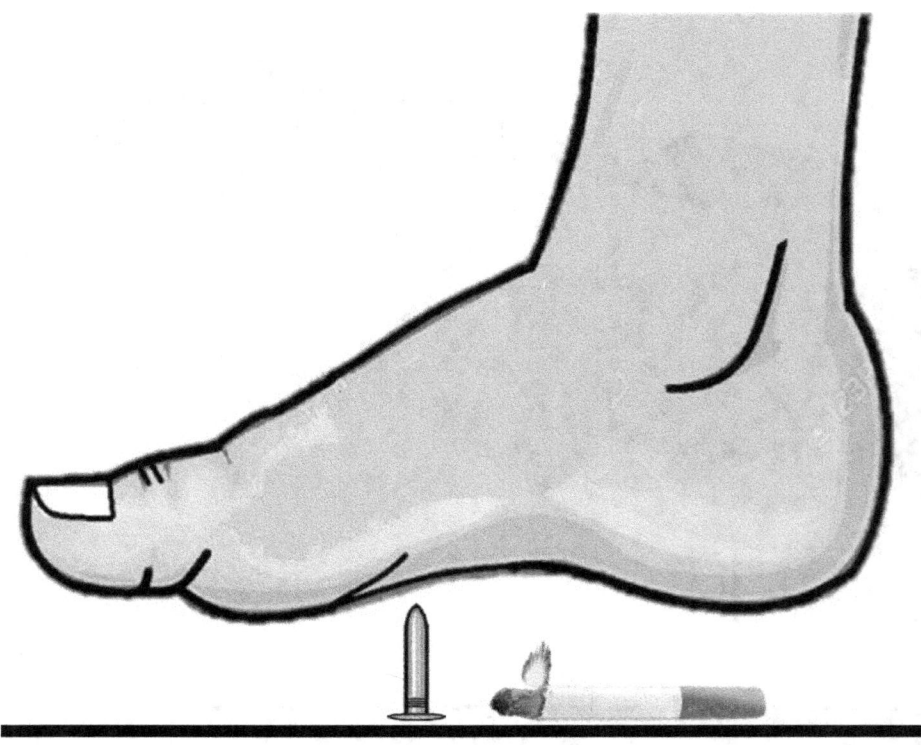

ADVISE #33
DO NOT WALK BAREFOOT IN ANY TYPE OF
SURFACE, A STUMBLE OR A FATAL
FOOTSTEP COULD BRING YOU SERIOUS
CONSEQUENCES TO THE FOOT.

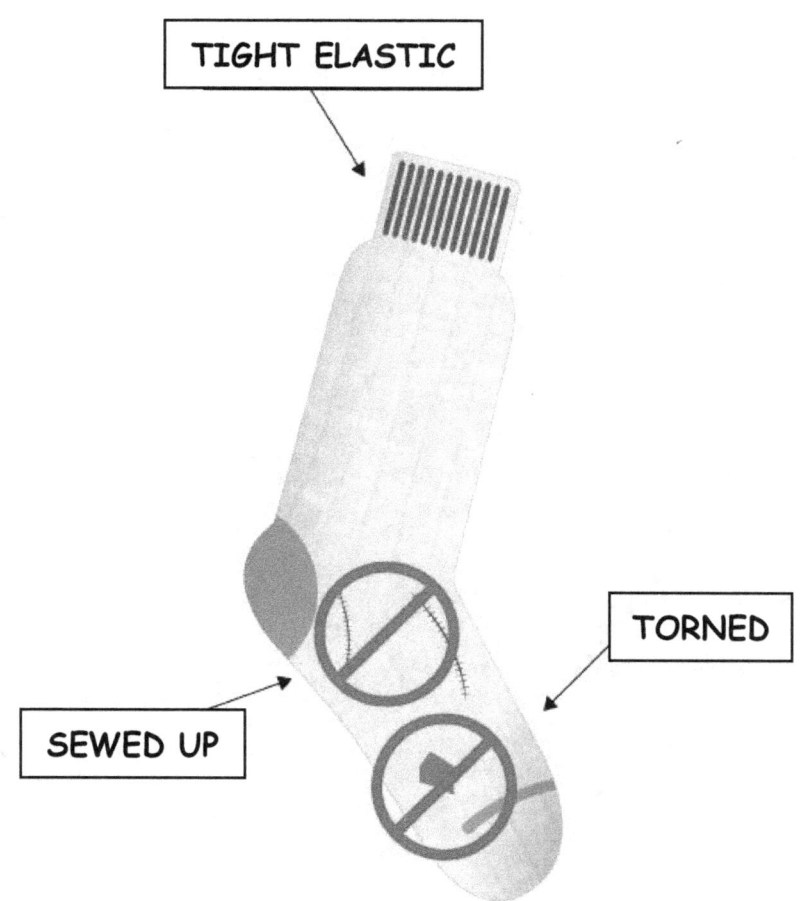

TIGHT ELASTIC

TORNED

SEWED UP

ADVICE #34
USE A PAIR OF CLEAN SOCKS EVERY DAY, WITHOUT HOLES, OR WITHOUT TIGHT ELASTIC AND DO NOT GET CRUSHED OR BENDED BY PUTTING THEM ON.
IF WHEN YOU REMOVE THEM, YOU NOTE A CIRCULAR SURFACE ON THE SKIN OF THE LEGS, GET RID OF THEM.

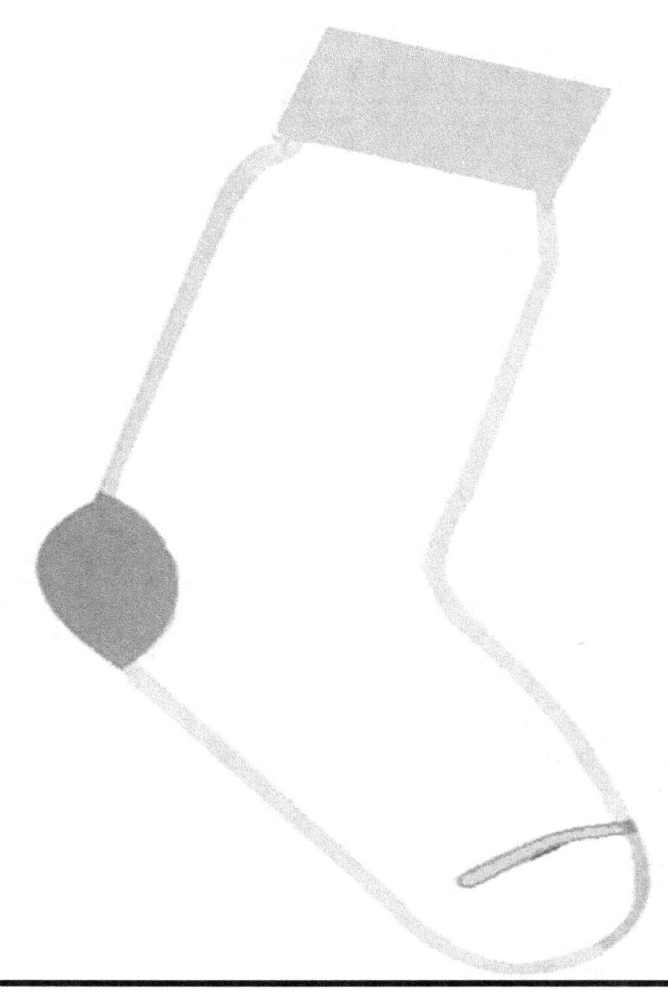

ADVICE #35

> USE SOCKS, PREFERABLY WHITE OR CLEAR TONES, OF WOOL, MADE OF THREAD OR COTTON. IF MIXED WITH SYNTHETIC MATERIAL, IT MUST BE IN A LOW PROPORTION.

> DO NOT USE SOCKS WHICH DISCOMFORT OR THAT IRRITATE THE SKIN.

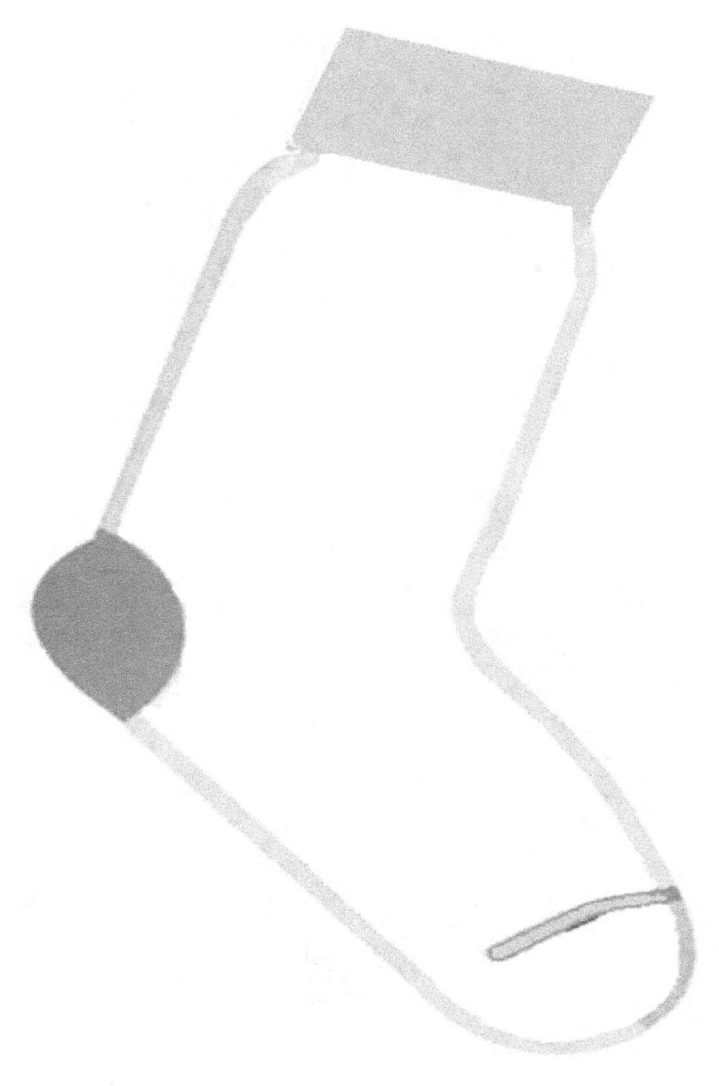

ADVICE #35. CONTINUACIÓN.
> SOCKS OF WOOL OR COTTON:
COLLECT THE SWEAT, ALLOW THE FEET TO
PERSPIRE AND MITIGATE THE FRICTION
WITH THE SHOE.

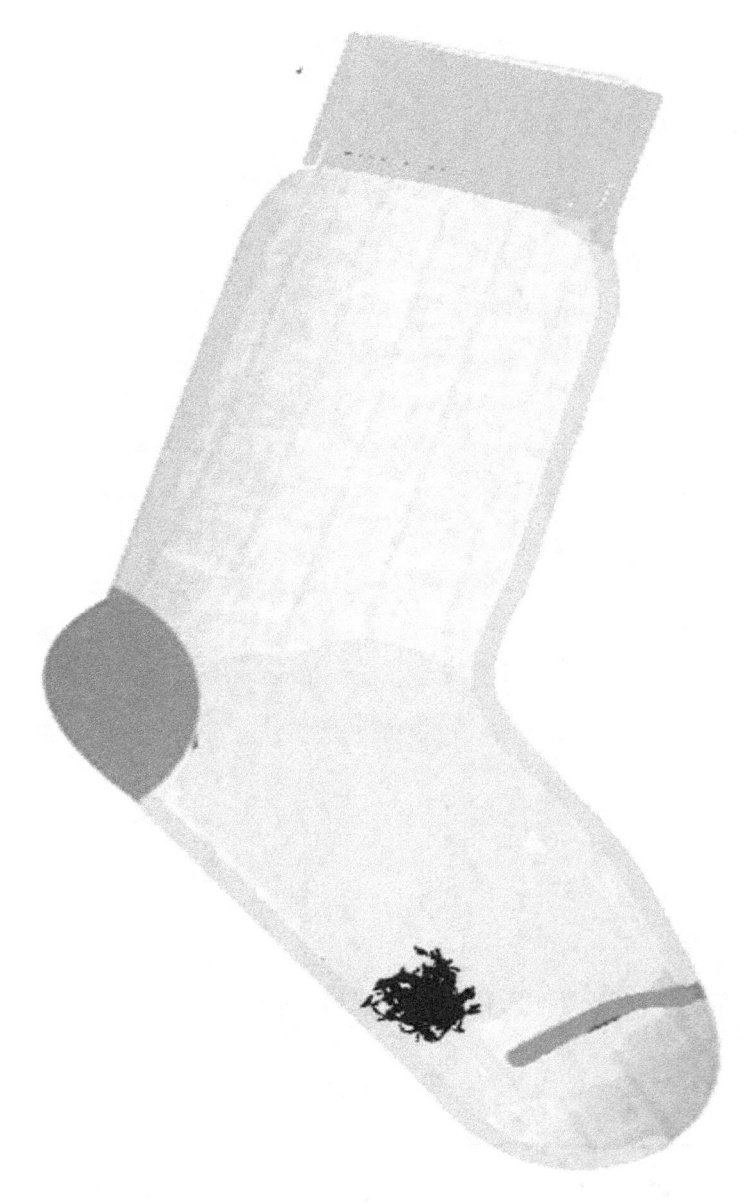

ADVICE #36
WHEN REMOVING SOCKS, CHECK THEM FOR
STAINS OF SOME LIQUID, BLOOD OR PUS.

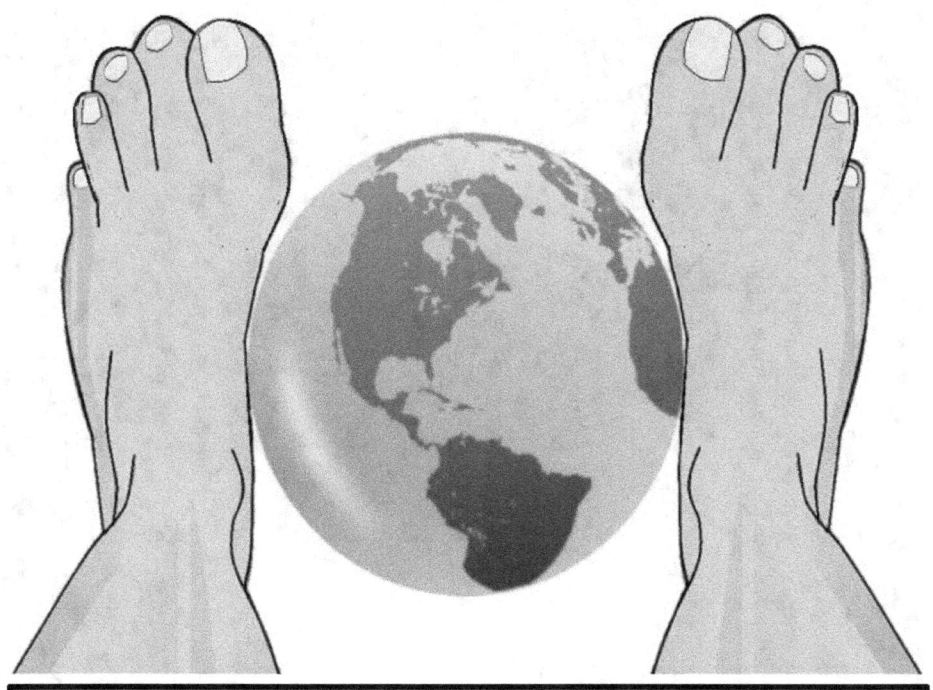

YOU NEED TO KNOW THE IMPORTANT
ASPECTS OF THE WORLD IN WHICH YOUR
FEET LIVE, THE POSSIBILITIES YOU
SHOULD LOSE THEM AND THE MULTIPLE
ADVICE TO AVOID THIS BODY DISASTER.

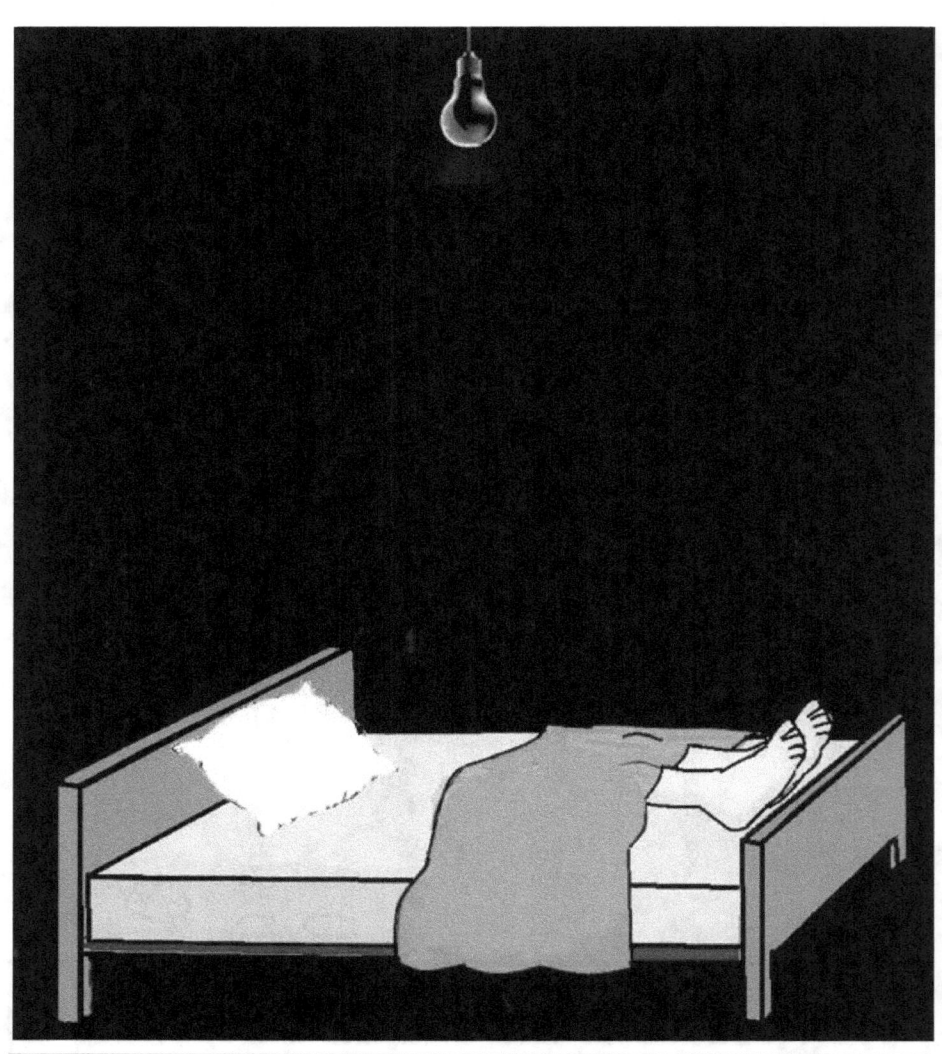

ADVICE #37
IF THE WEATHER ALLOW YOU, SLEEP
WITHOUT SOCKS SO YOUR FEET CAN
BREATHE FREELY.

ELECTRIC
BLANKET

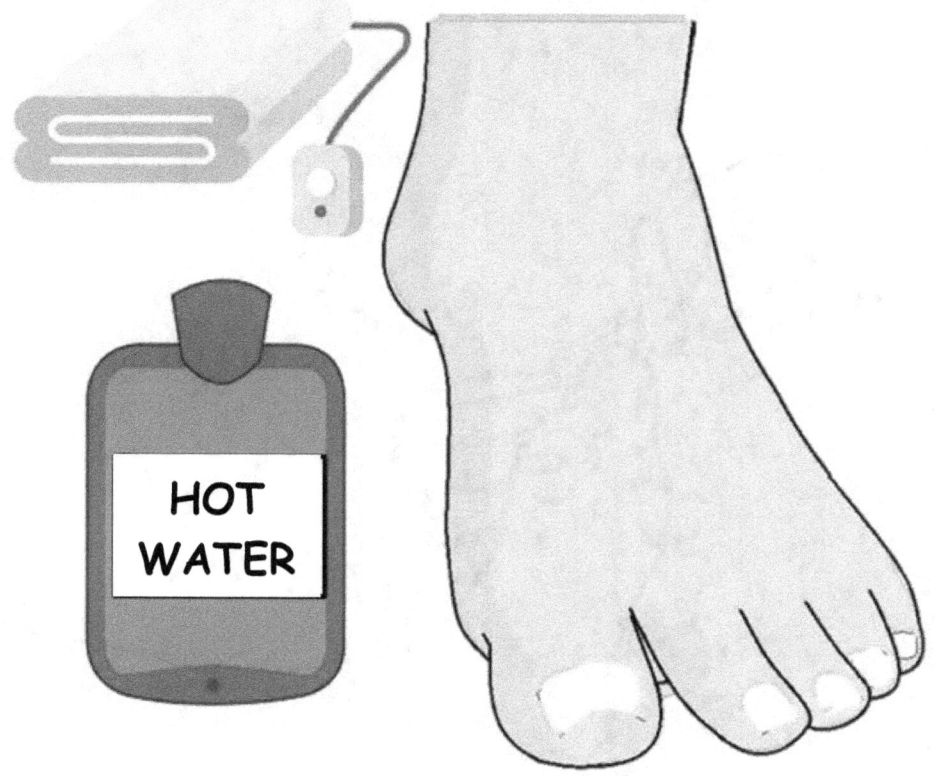

HOT
WATER

ADVICE #38
> DO NOT APPLY EXTERNAL HEAT IN THE
FOOT OR STAY NEAR ELEMENTS THAT
DIFFUSE HIGH TEMPERATURE: ELECTRIC
HEATERS, CHIMNEYS, FIREPLACES. YOU
MAY CAUSE A BURN.

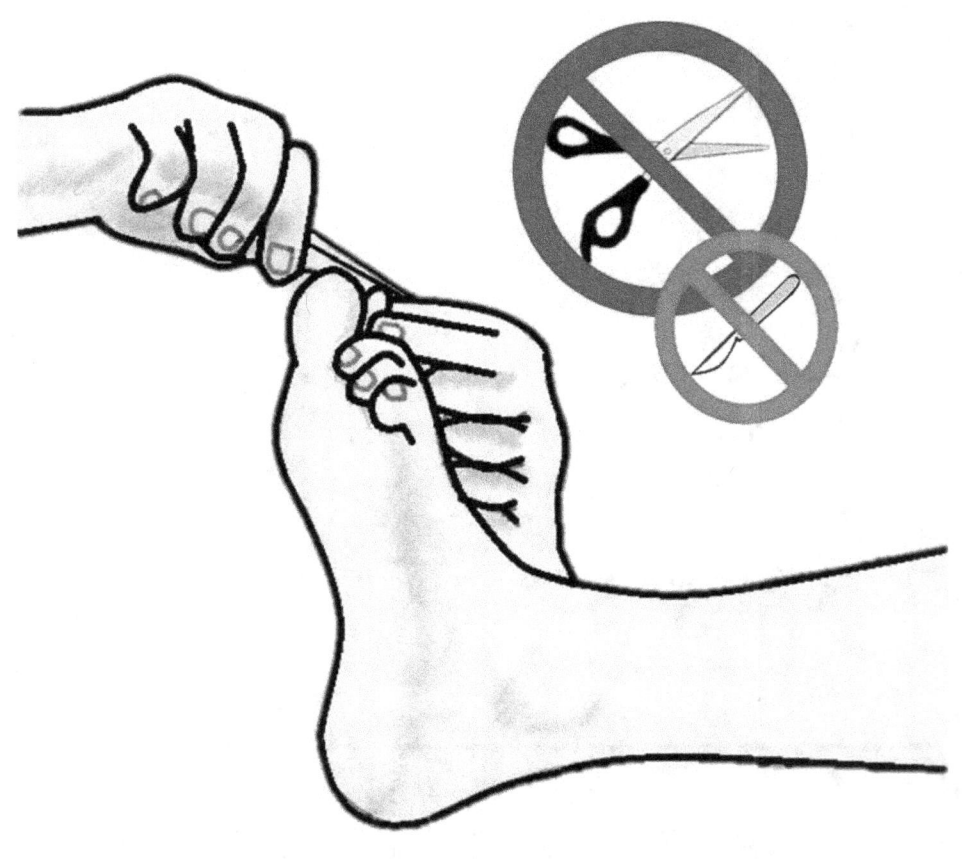

ADVICE #39
> DO NOT DO "HOME SURGERY" ON INGROWN NAILS, CALLOSITIES OR IN THE CALLUS.

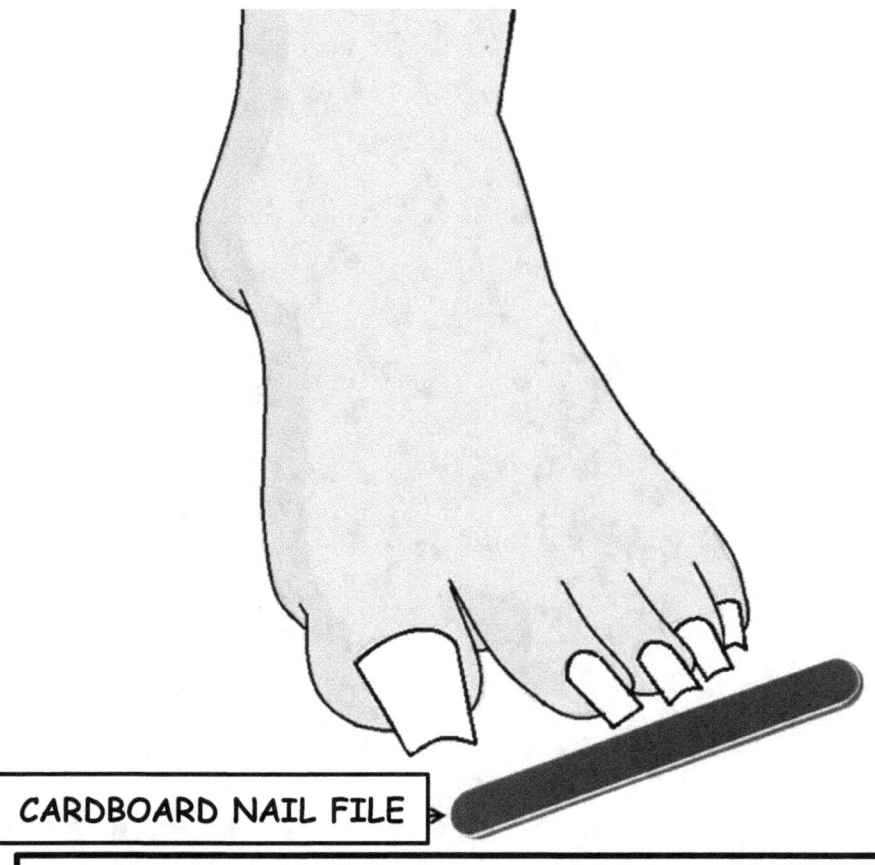

CARDBOARD NAIL FILE

ADVICE #40
> THE NAILS SHOULD BE CUT BY A
PODIATRIC AND WARN HIM THAT YOU ARE
DIABETIC AND DO NOT CUT THE NAILS
TOO SHORT ON THE POINTS OR THE
ANGLES, IT COULD BURRIED AND BECOME
INFECTED (INGROWN TOENAILS).
> IF YOU WOULD LIKE TO REDUCE IT
PROVISIONALLY, USE A CARDBOARD
NAILS.

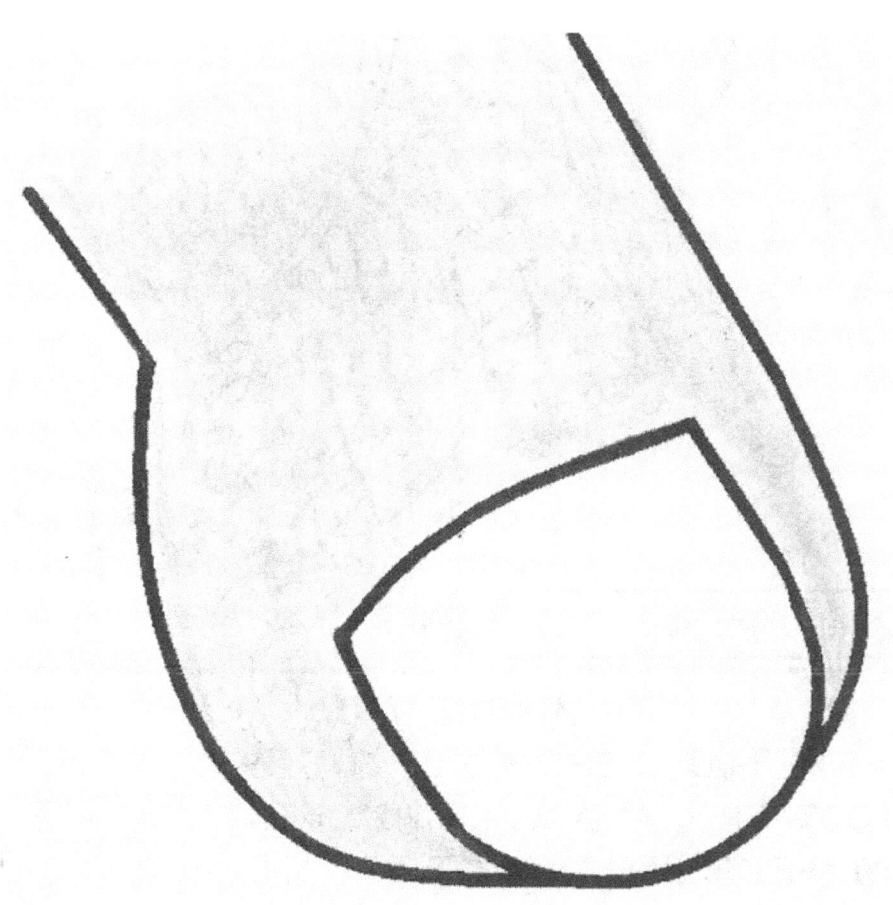

ADVICE #41. CONTINUATION.
DO NOT LEAVE THE CORNERS OF THE NAIL
SHARP POINTED OR SHARP NAILS, IT IS
BETTER TO SMOOTH THEM A BIT TO MAKE
THEM BLUNT.

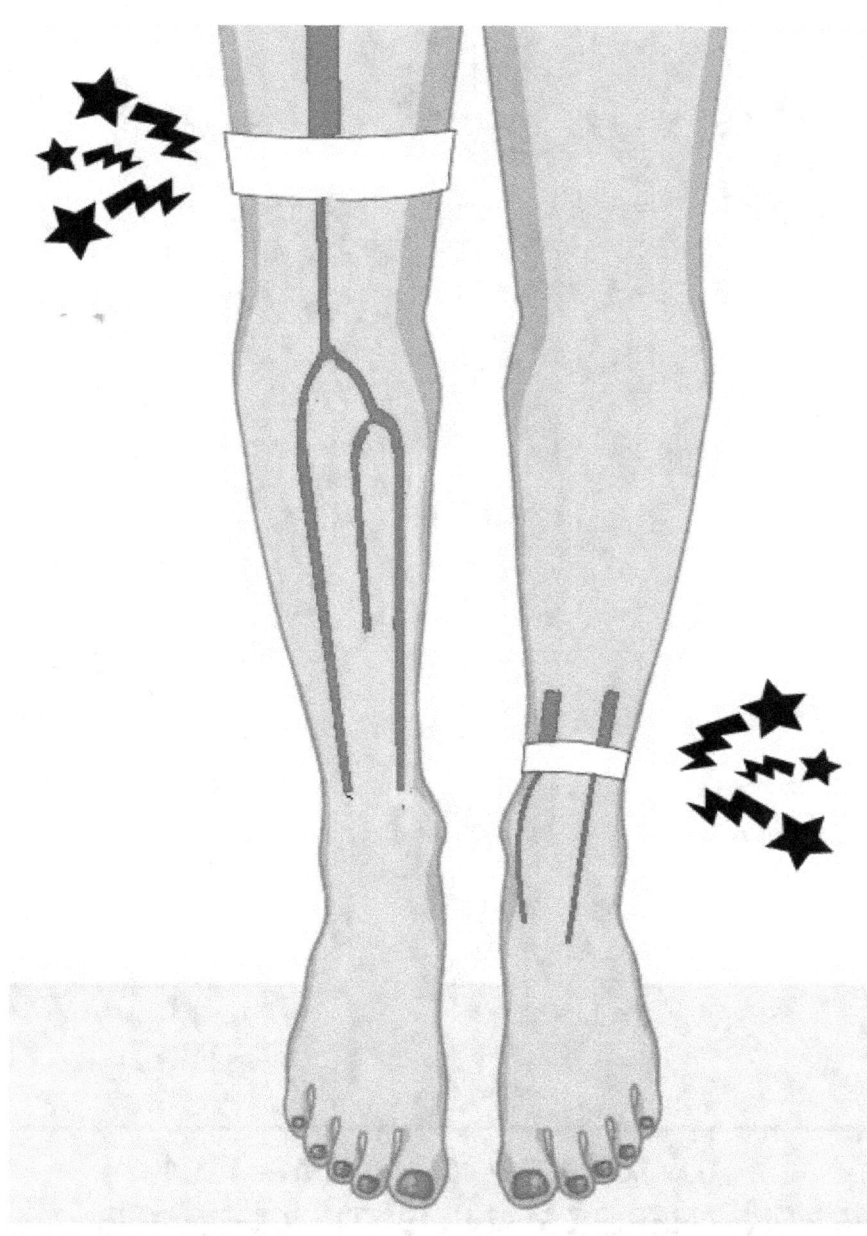

ADVICE #42
DO NOT USE SUSPENDERS OR SOCKS THAT
TIGHTEN YOUR SKIN AND DIFFICULT THE
BLOOD CIRCULATION IN THE FEET.

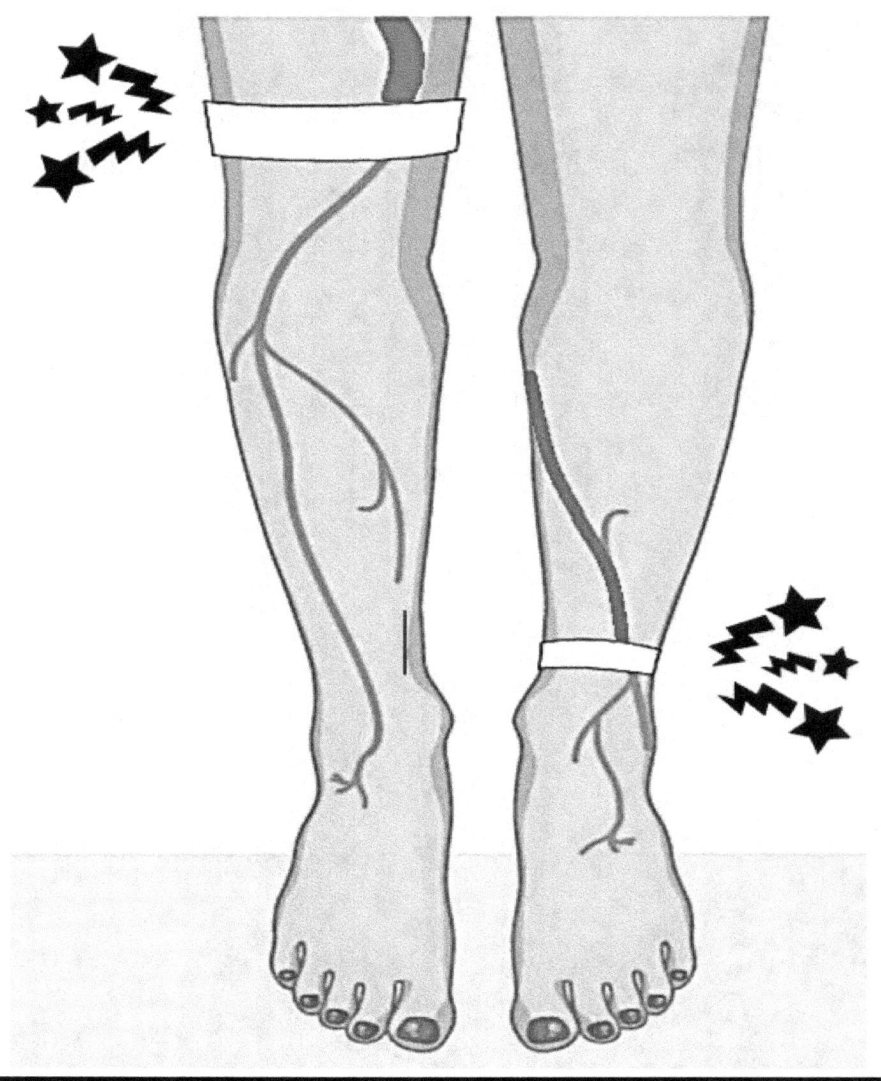

ADVICE #42. CONTINUATION.
WHEN THERE IS AN OBSTRUCTED DEEP
ARTERY, THE BODY TENDS TO
COMPENSATE FOR THE LACK OF DISTAL
BLOOD WITH SMALL SURFACE ARTERIES
(COLLATERAL CIRCULATION).

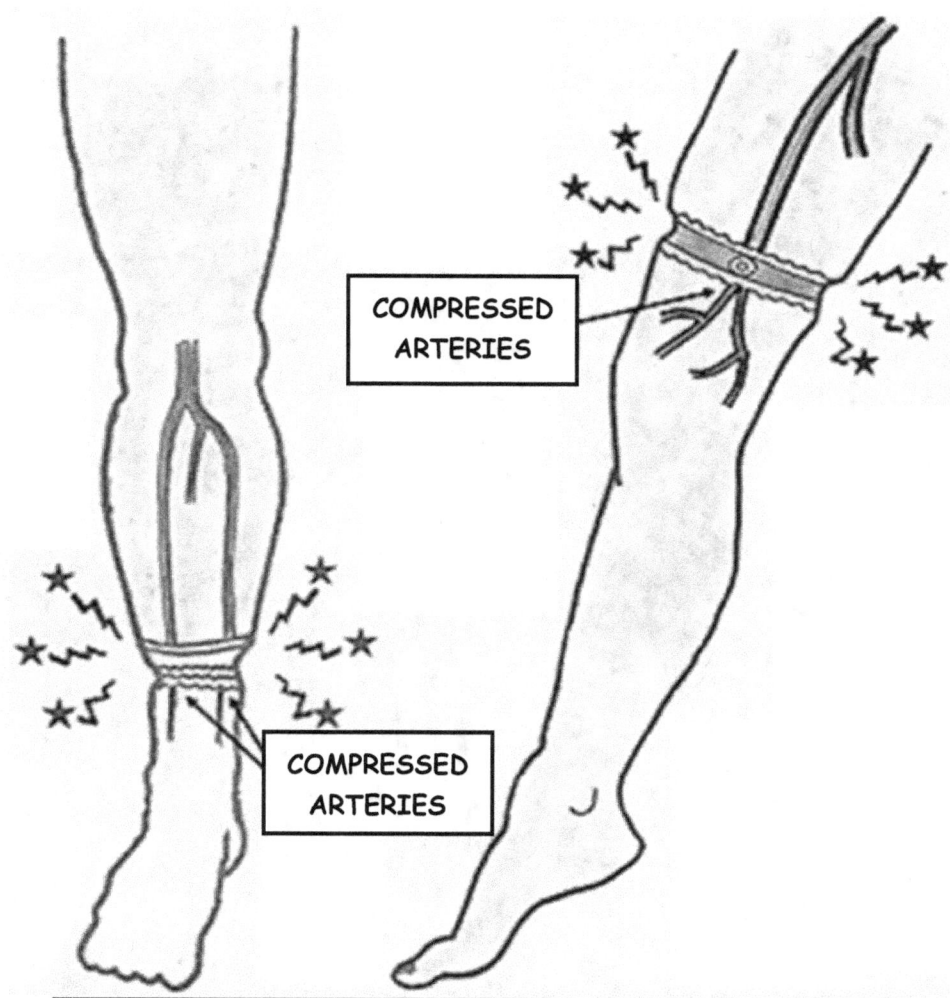

COMPRESSED
ARTERIES

COMPRESSED
ARTERIES

ADVICE #42. CONTINUATION.
> THESE SMALL ARTERIES ARE THOSE
THAT CAN BE COMPRESSED AND DISTAL
BLOOD FAILURE IS INCREASED.
> THE DECREASE OF ARTERIAL BLOOD
FLOW CONTRIBUTES TO THE
APPEARANCE OF COMPLICATIONS.

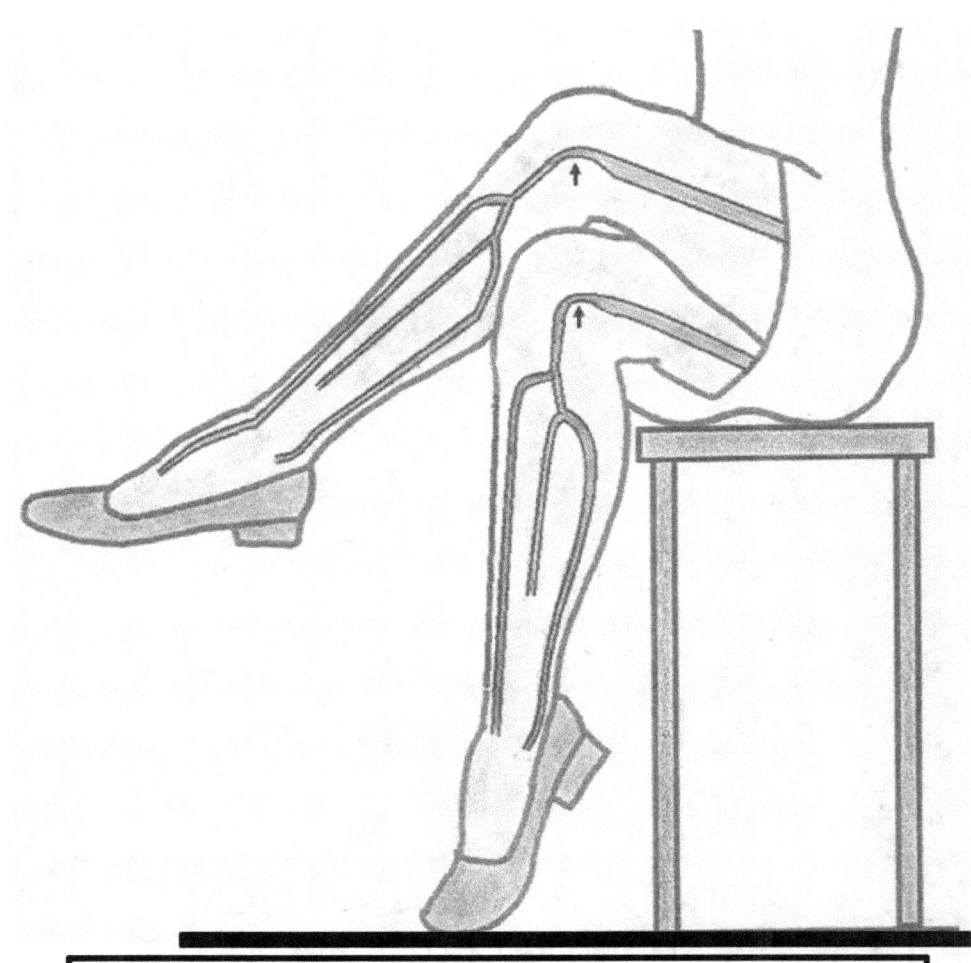

ADVICE #43
DO NOT SEAT WITH CROSSED LEGS OR KNEES FOR A PROLONGED PERIOD, THIS POSITION SLOWS DOWN THE BLOOD CIRCULATION TO THE FEET.

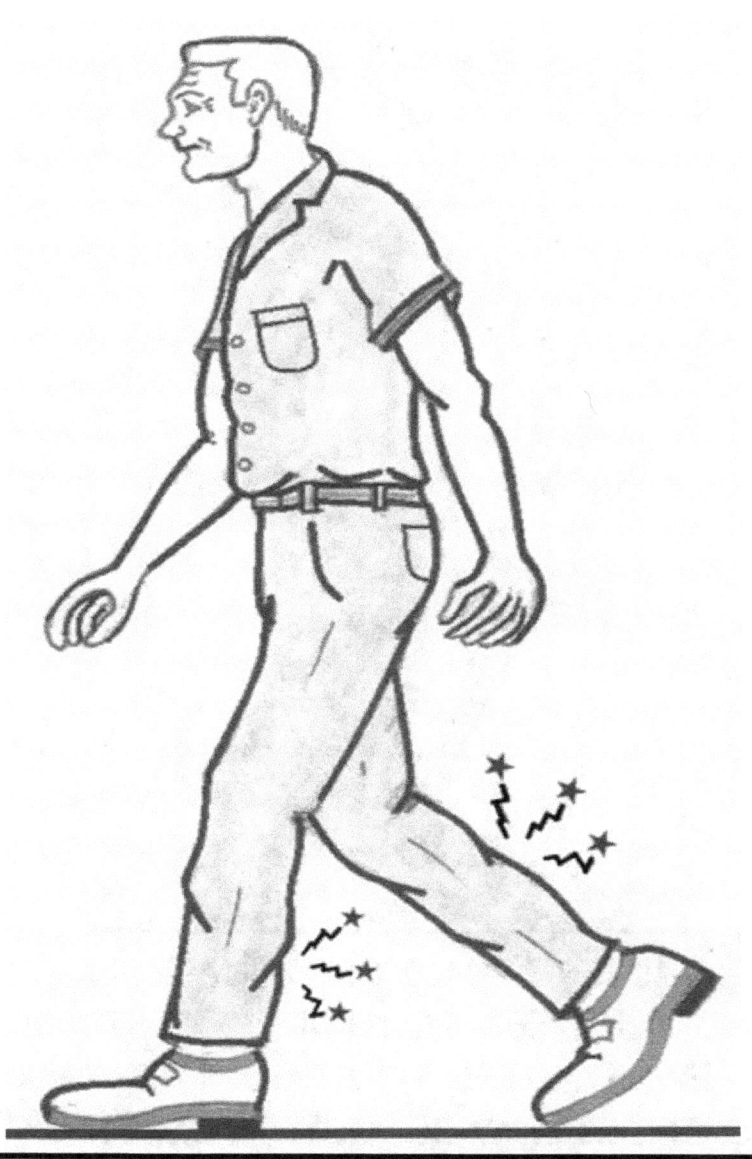

ADVICE #44
IF WHEN YOU WALK A SHORT
DISTANCE (HALF OR ONE BLOCK) YOU
FEEL PAIN OR CRAMPS IN THE
MUSCULAR MASSES OF YOUR LEGS,

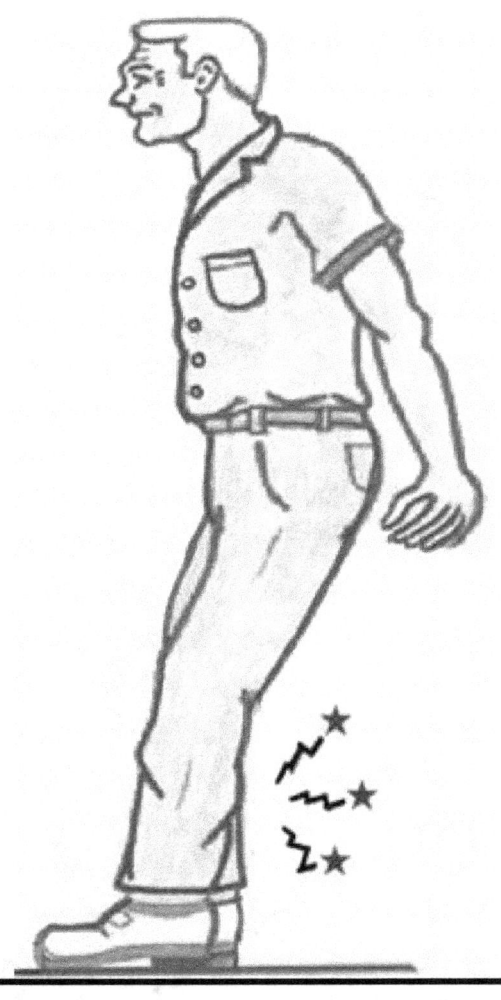

ADVICE #44. CONTINUATION.
AND YOU NEED TO STOP TO REST FOR
A FEW MINUTES TO START THE WALK
AGAIN, IT MAY BE A SYMPTOM OF
NARROWING OR OCLUSION OF THE
ARTERIES THAT BRING BLOOD TO YOUR
FEET.
CONSULT YOUR PRIMARY PHYSICIAN
AND EXPLAIN YOUR SYMPTOMS.

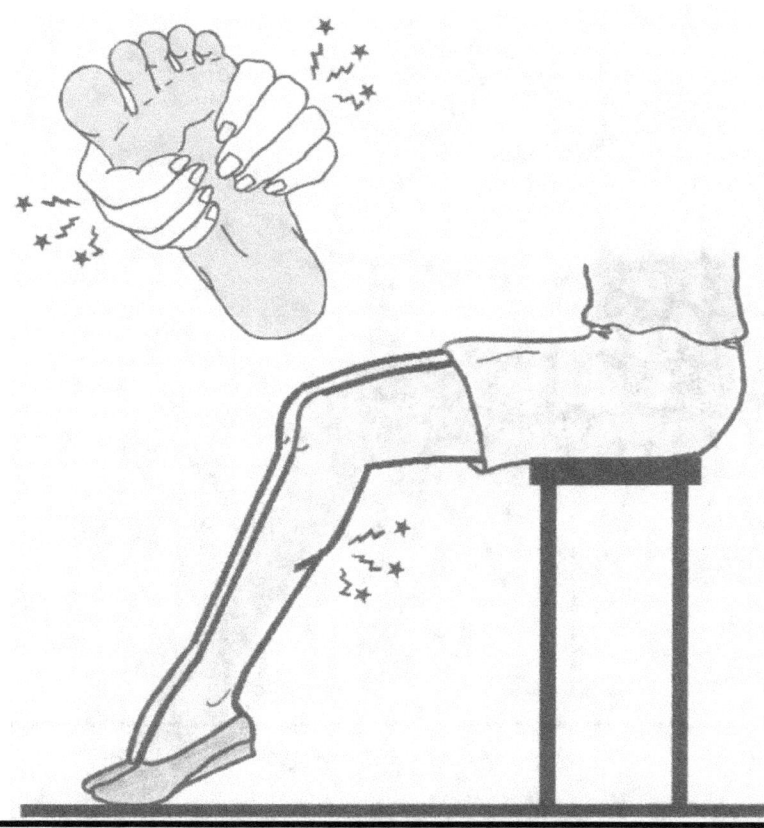

ADVICE #45

> IF YOU HAVE PAIN IN THE MUSCULAR MASSES OF THE LEGS OR FEET AT REST, NOT RELIEVED WITH THE ANALGESICS INDICATED BY YOUR PHYSICIAN, IT MAY BE A TOTAL OCLUSION (TROMBOSIS) OF THE ARTERIES THAT IRRIGATE YOUR LEGS.
> REQUEST AN APPOINTMENT WITH THE PRIMARY PHYSICIAN AND EXPLAIN YOUR SYMPTOMS.

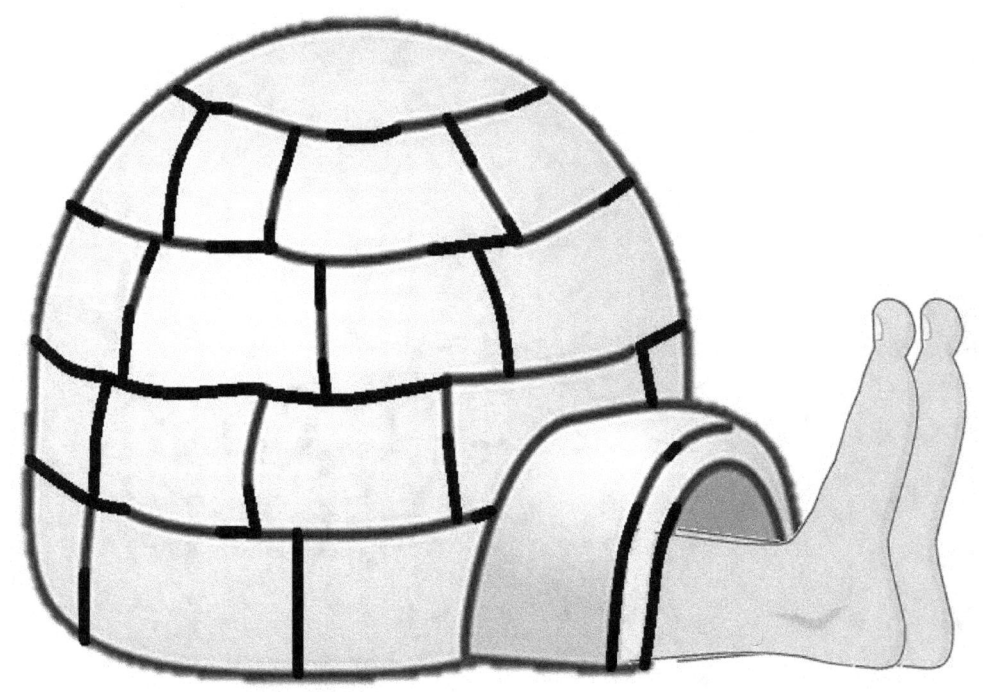

ADVICE #46

> PROTECT YOUR FEET FROM THE COLD, ESPECIALLY IF YOU HAVE ARTERIAL DISEASE, BECAUSE IT CAN CAUSE A SPASM OF THE ARTERIES OF YOUR LEGS AND CAN CAUSE THE DEATH OF TISSUES OR "FREEZING GANGRENE" AT YOUR FEET.
> DURING THE WINTER USE SOCKS MADE OF WOOL AND COVERED SHOES, AND BLANKETS TO COVER THEM IN THE EVENING, IN ADDITION TO THE HEATING OF THE HOUSE TO AVOID THIS COMPLICATION.

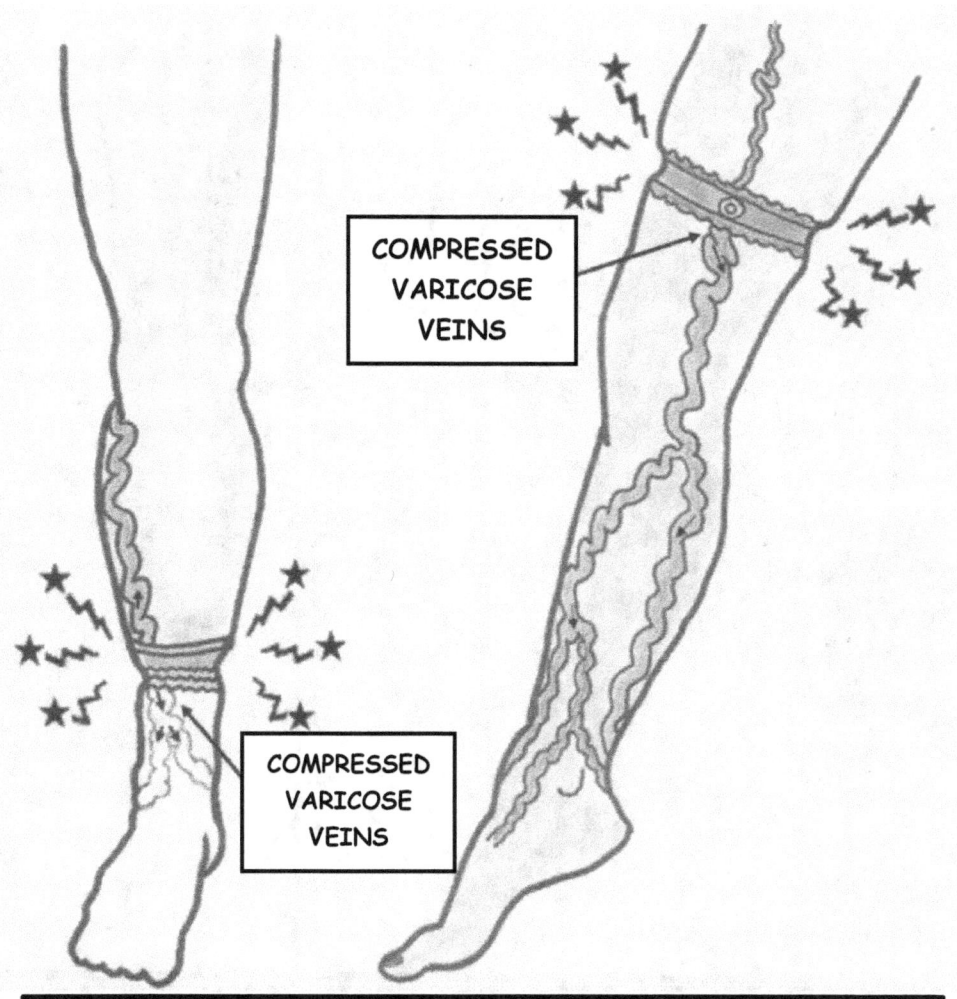

COMPRESSED
VARICOSE
VEINS

COMPRESSED
VARICOSE
VEINS

ADVICE #47

IF YOU ARE DIABETIC AND HAVE VARICOSE
VEINS, DO NOT USE SOCKS WITH
ELASTICS THAT TIGHTEN YOUR SKIN'S
TISSUES AND STRAIN THE CIRCULATION
THAT DRAINS VENOUS BLOOD FROM THE
FEET IN THE HEART AND MAKES THE
APPEARANCE OF A COMPLICATION.

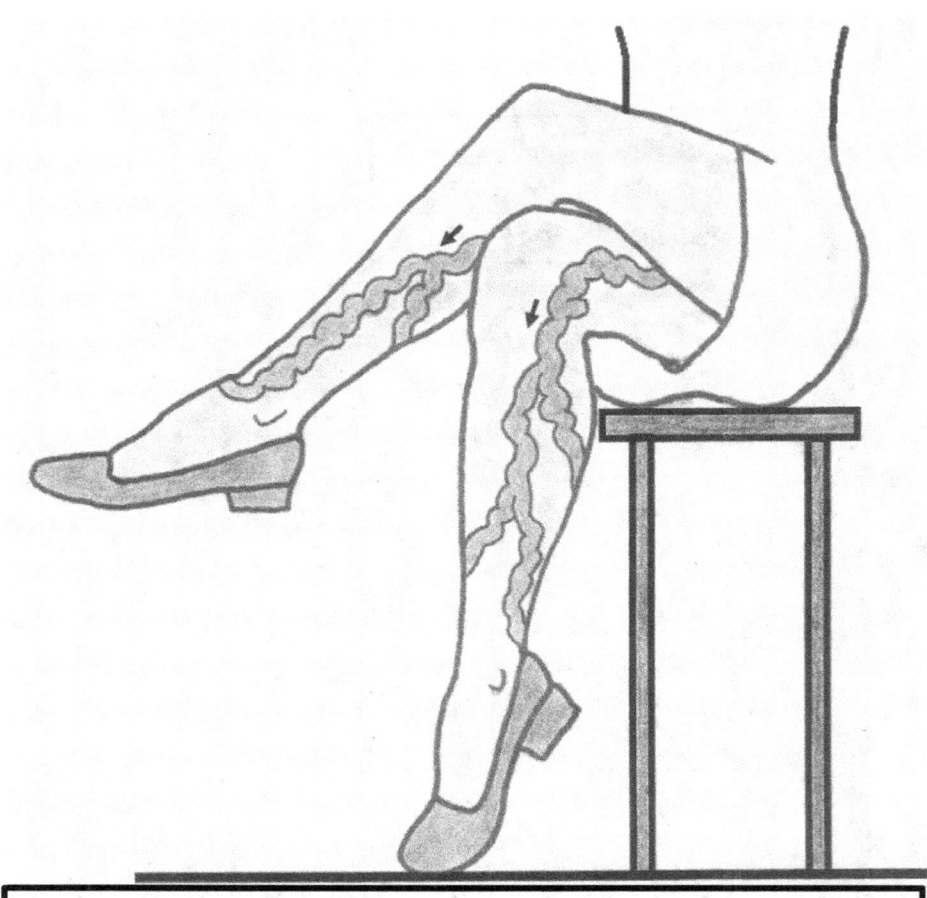

ADVICE #48
IF IN ADDITION TO BEING DIABETIC, THE PATIENT HAS VARICOSE VEINS, DO NOT SEAT WITH THE CROSSED LEGS OR KNEES A LONG PERIOD OF TIME, THIS POSITION INCREASES THE SLOW DOWN VENOUS CIRCULATION IN THE FEET AND FAVORS A COMPLICATION.

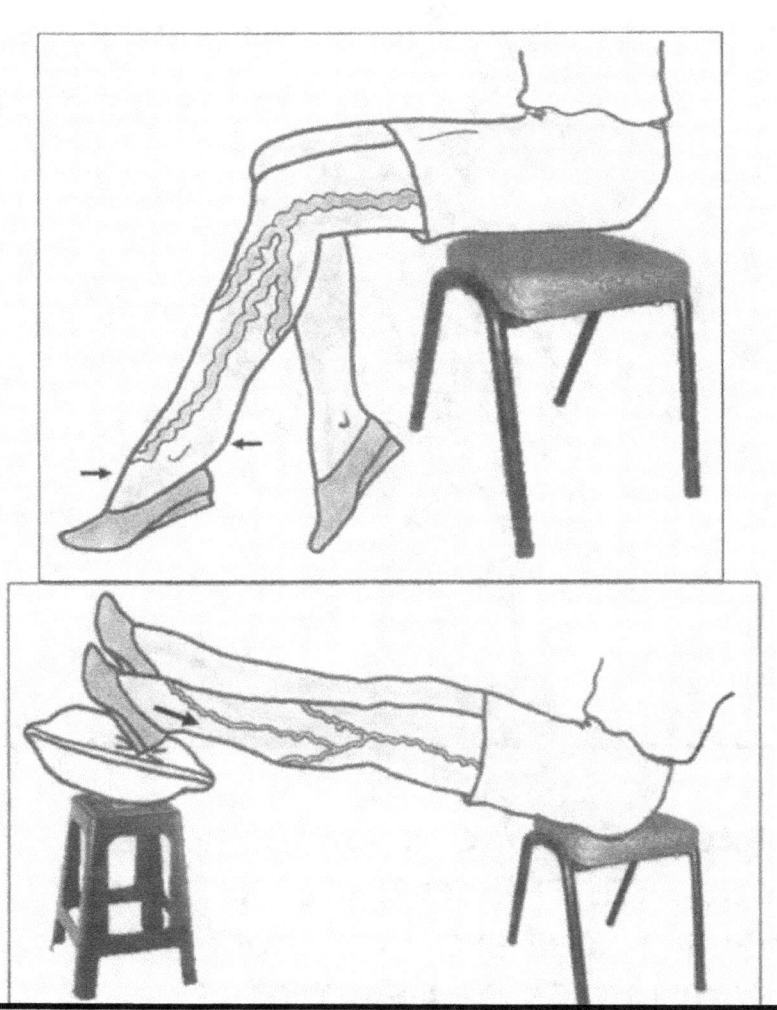

ADVICE #49

IF YOU ARE DIABETIC AND HAVE INCREASED VOLUME OF THE FOOT AND/OR VARICOSE VEINS, WHEN YOU ARE SITTING, PUT IT WITHOUT A SHOE ON A TABLE AND SUPPORT UP A PILLOW OR PAD TO FACILITATE THE DRAINING OF THE ACCUMULATED LIQUID.

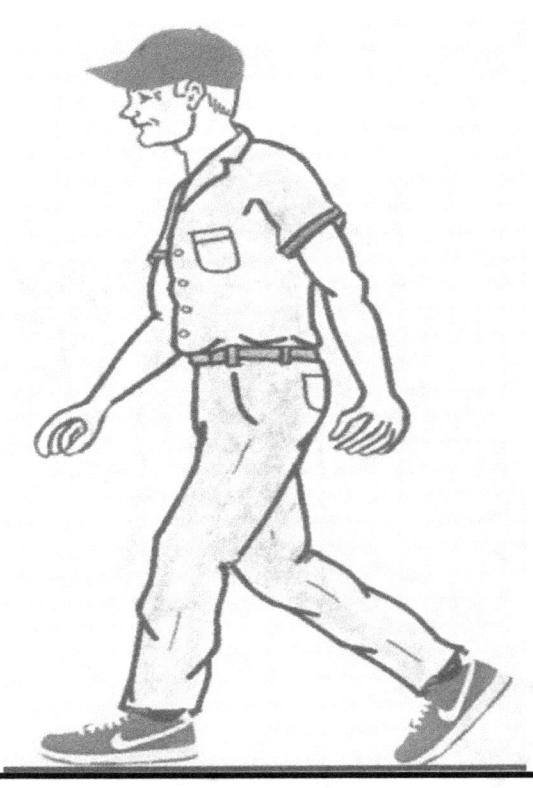

ADVICE #50
> PRACTICE ANY KIND OF EXERCISE, FACILITATE THE CONTROL OF SUGAR LEVELS IN THE BLOOD, REDUCE THE POSSIBILITIES OF HEART DISEASE, MAINTAIN A GENERAL WELL-BEING STATE AND IMPROVE THE CIRCULATION IN YOUR LEGS, DECREASING THE POSSIBILITY OF HAVING A COMPLICATION THAT NEED AN AMPUTATION.
> RECOMMENDED EXERCISES: WALKING, CALLISTHENICS, SWIMMING AND STATIONARY BICYCLE.

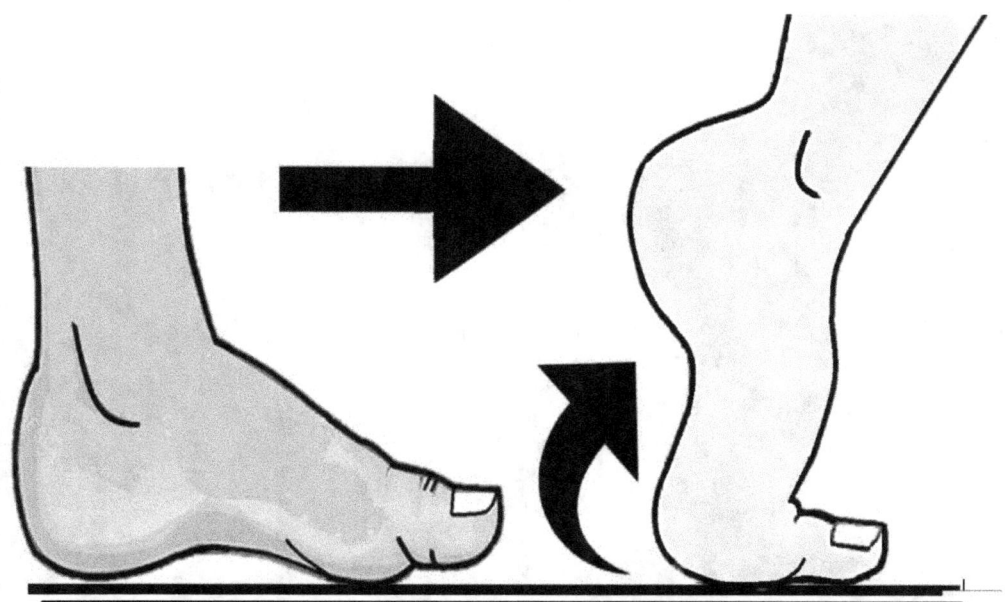

ADVICE #50. EXERCISES, CONTINUED.
ALL EXERCISES WE RECOMMEND MUST BE
AUTHORIZED BY A PHYSICIAN IN
DEPENDENCE OF YOUR AGE, EXISTING
DISEASES AND PHYSICAL LIMITATIONS
AND INDICATED AND SUPERVISED BY A
PHYSIOTHERAPIST.
THE FOLLOWING ARE ALSO USEFUL TO
IMPROVE THE CIRCULATION OF THE FEET:
STAND UP ON THE POINT OF THE FEET
REPEATEDLY.

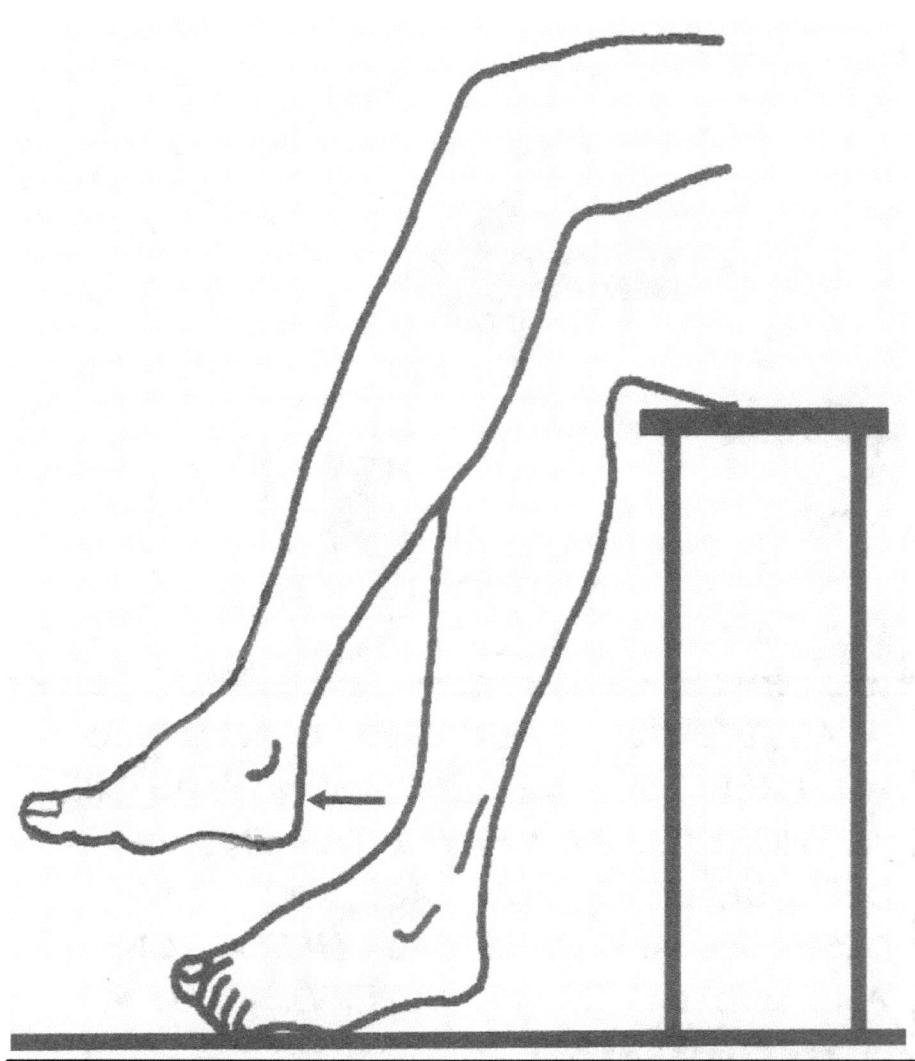

ADVICE #50. EXERCISES, CONTINUED. PLACE THE FOOT WHICH YOU WANT TO EXERCISE FIRST IN A HORIZONTAL POSITION.

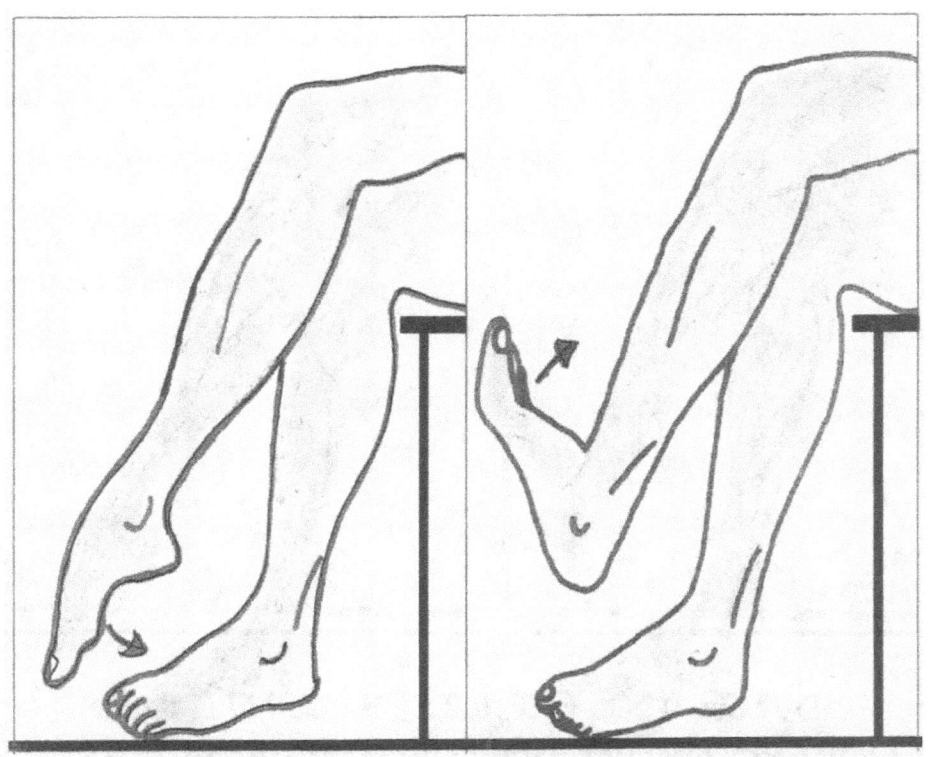

ADVICE #50. EXERCISES, CONTINUED.
> MOVE THEM DOWN (EXTENSION) AND UP
(FLEXION) VARIOUS TIMES.
> THIS EXERCISE SHOULD BE APPROVED BY
YOUR PRIMARY PHYSICIAN OR QUALIFIED
PERSONNEL TO DETERMINE THE NUMBER
OF TIMES YOU MUST DO IT.

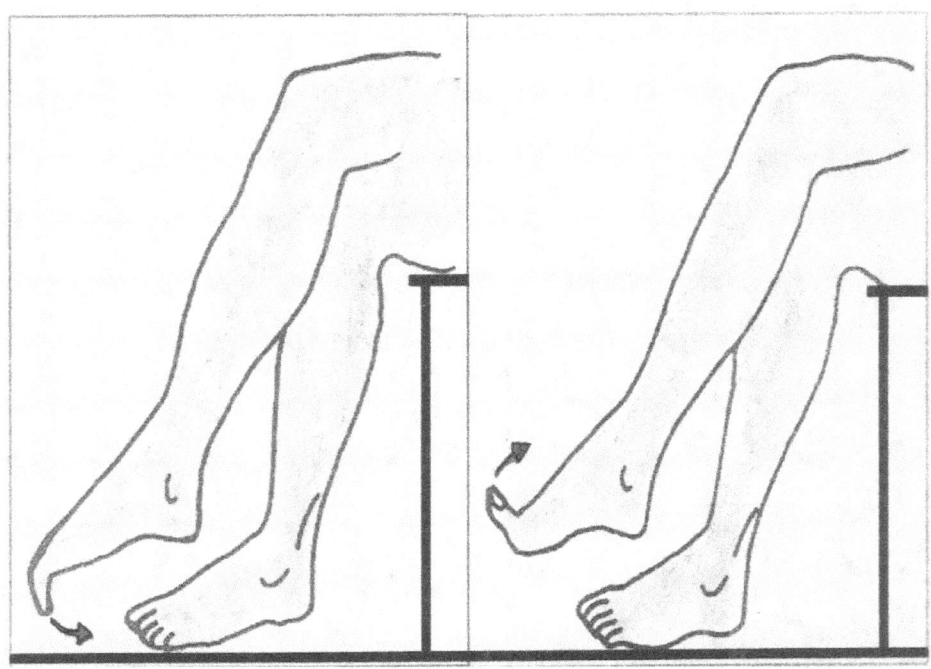

ADVICE #50. EXERCISES, CONTINUED. NOW YOU MUST DO THE SAME EXERCISE WITH THE TOES OF THE FOOT:
> MOVE THEM DOWN (EXTENSION) AND UP (FLEXION) REPEATLY.
> THIS EXERCISE SHOULD BE AUTHORIZED BY YOUR ASSISTANCE PHYSICIAN OR A QUALIFIED PERSONNEL TO DETERMINE THE NUMBER OF TIMES YOU MUST DO.

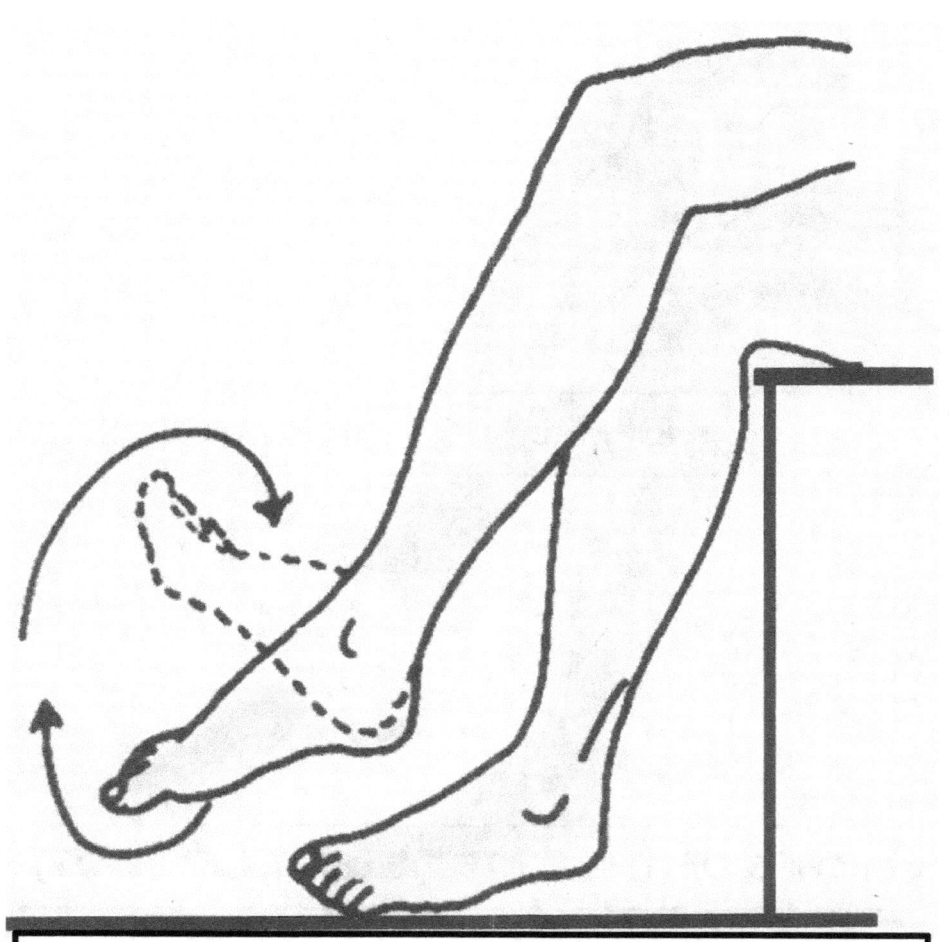

ADVICE #50. EXERCISES, FINAL.
> PERFORM A CIRCULAR MOVEMENT IN BOTH DIRECTIONS, FROM RIGHT TO LEFT AND FROM LEFT TO RIGHT.
> THIS EXERCISE SHOULD BE APPROVED BY YOUR ASSISTANCE PHYSICIAN OR A QUALIFIED PERSONNEL WHO WILL DETERMINE THE NUMBER OF TIMES YOU MUST DO.

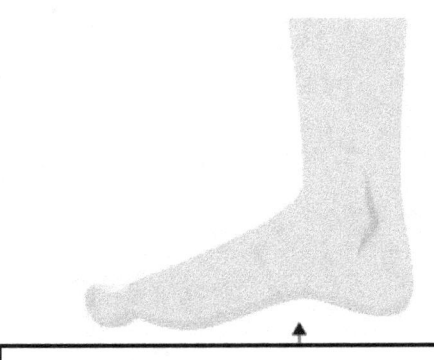

NORMAL FOOT ARCHES

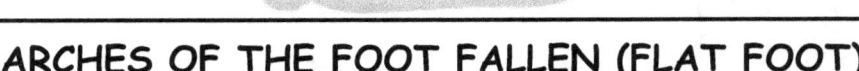

ARCHES OF THE FOOT FALLEN (FLAT FOOT)

ADVICE #51

IF YOU OBSERVE THAT THE ARCHES OF THE FOOT (TRANSVERSE OR LONGITUDINAL) ARE FALLEN (FLAT FOOT) OR ANY OTHER DEFORMITIES OF THE FOOT, PLEASE CONSULT THE ORTHOPEDIST OR PODIATRIST TO CORRECT THE DEFECT WITH ORTHOPEDIC SHOES OR SOLE SUPPORTS AND AVOID A CORN OR CALLUS FORMING.

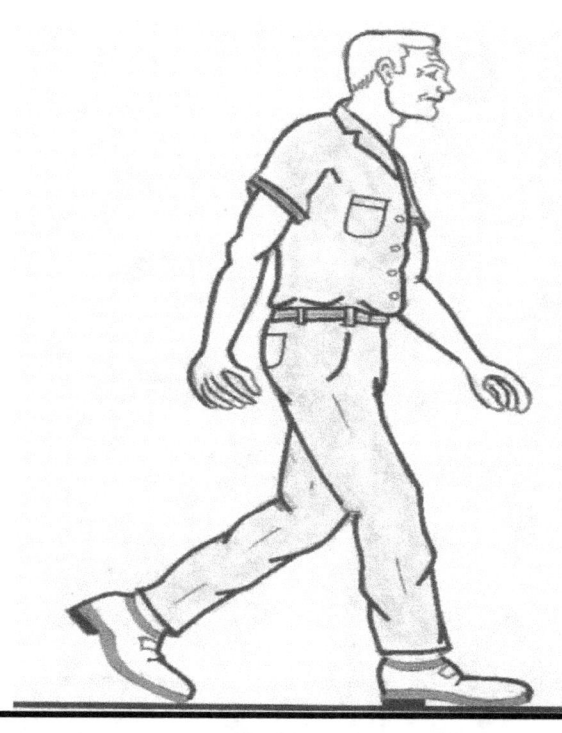

ADVICE #52

IF YOU PERCIVE A CHANGE IN THE
MECHANICS OF YOUR WALK AND THIS
ACCOMPANIES ANY FOOT DEFORMITY,
DISORDERS TO MOBILIZE THEM AND HAVE
SYMPTOMS OF ARTHRITIS (PAIN) ON THE
FOOT, ANKLE OR KNEE, ASK THE PRIMARY
PHYSICIAN AN APPOINTMENT WITH THE
PODOLOGIST TO CORRECTS DEFECTS OF
THE FOOT TO IMPROVE YOUR
DEAMBULATION AND AVOID THE
FORMATION OF A CALLOSITY AND
POSSIBLE ULCERATION.

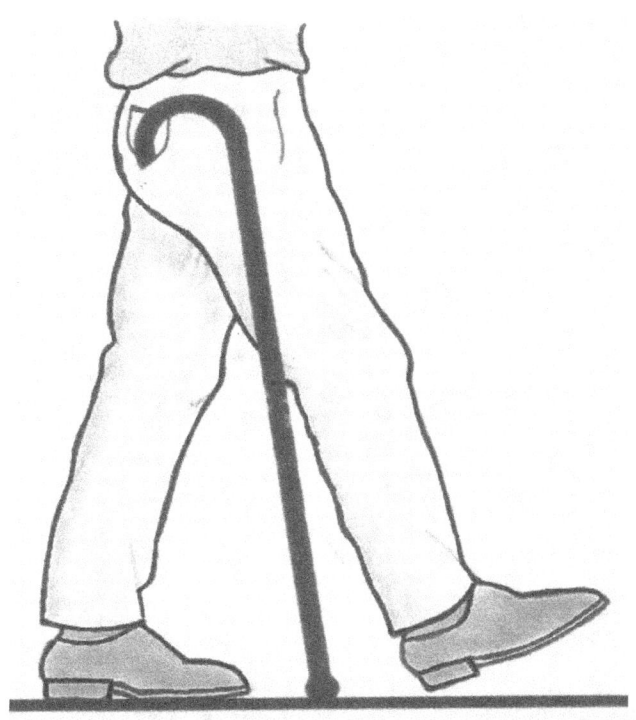

ADVICE #52. CONTINUATION

> THE PODOLOGIST WILL MAKE DIFFERENT STUDIES TO DETERMINE THE DEVICE TO USE TO CORRECT THE EXISTING DEFECTS AND RESTORE THE LOST FUNCTIONS TO THE NEAREST NORMALITY.

> POSSIBLE RESOURCES TO BE USED: ORTHOPEDIC SHOES, SUPPORTS, SEPARATORS OF FINGERS, RINGS AND FUNDS OF FINGERS, PROTECTORS AND CORRECTORS OF BUNIONS.

> YOU MAY NEED TO USE A CANE OR A WALKER.

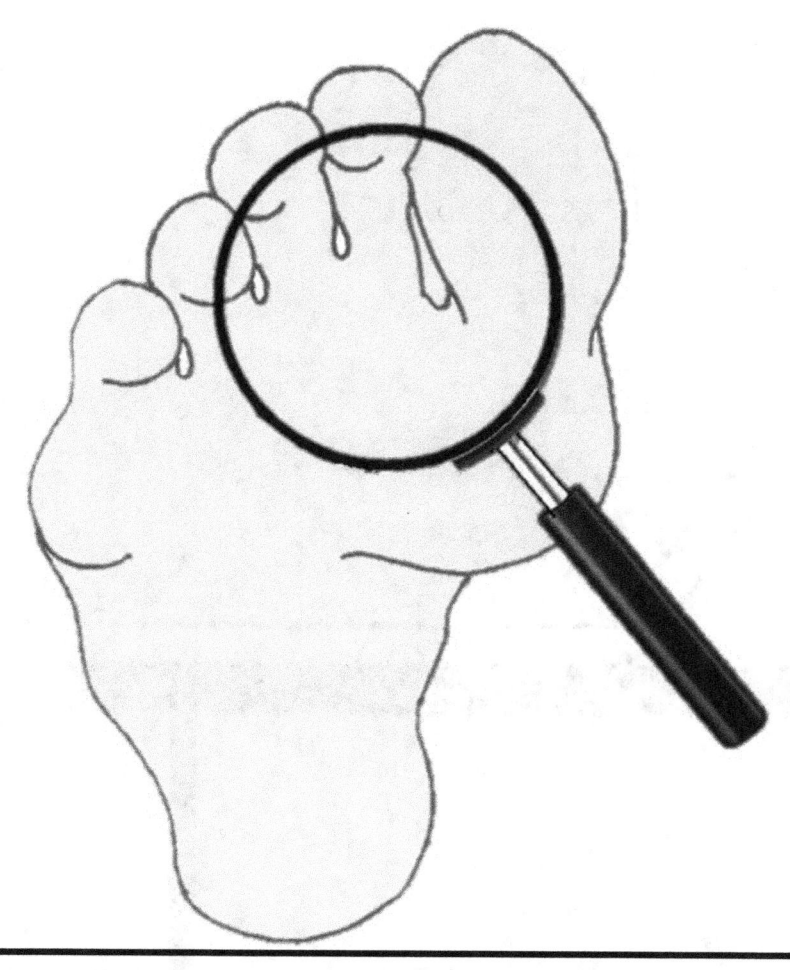

REMEMBER THAT YOU MUST PAY
ATTENTION TO THE MOST MINIMAL
DETAILS OF THE EVERYDAY LIFE OF YOUR
FEET TO ACHIEVE THEIR SURVIVAL, SINCE
THEY LIVE THEIR EVENTS THAT MAY
APPEAR INSIGNIFICANT, BUT THEY
ACQUIRE IMPORTANCE WHEN EVENTS CAN
DETERMINE THEIR FINAL DESTINY.

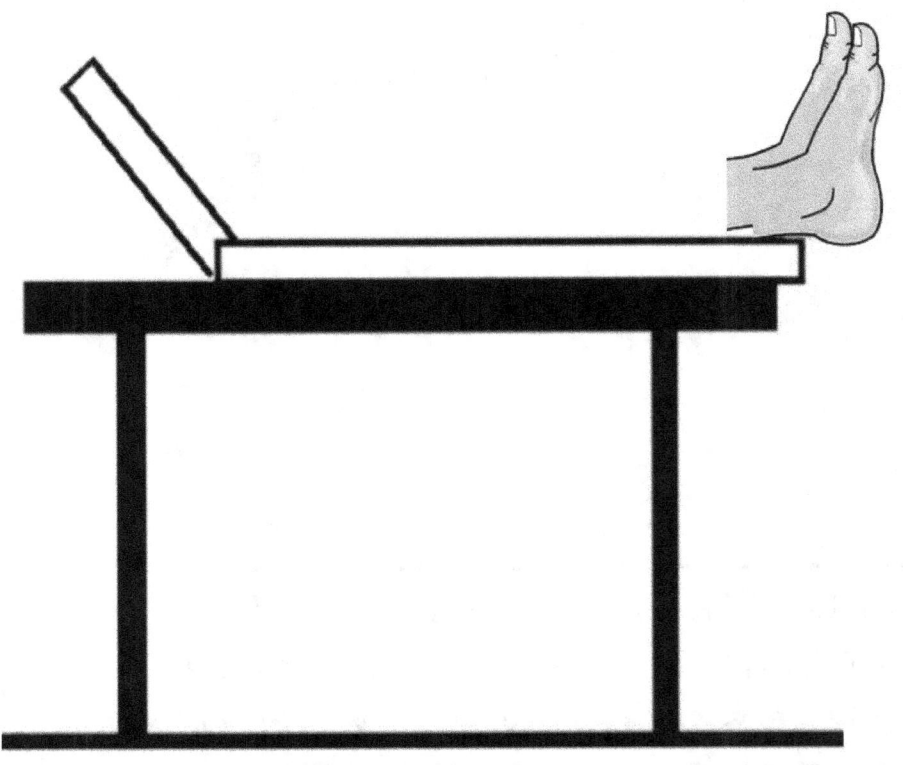

ADVICE #53
WHEN YOU HAVE A DOCTOR'S
APPOINTMENT, TAKE OFF YOUR SHOES
AND SOCKS, SHOW YOUR FEET AND ASK
HIM TO EXAMINE THEM.

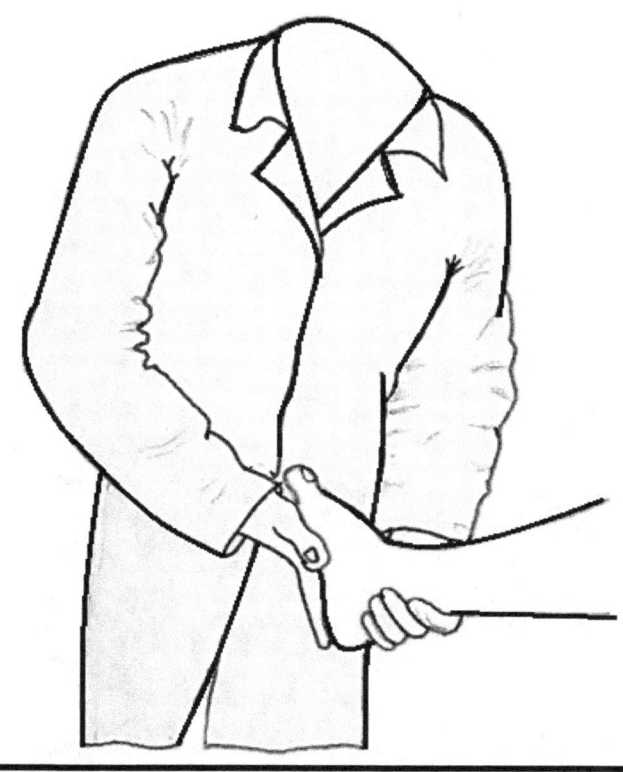

ADVICE #54

> PLEASE CONSULT WITH YOUR PRIMARY PHYSICIAN OR THE PODIATRIST EVERY SIX MONTHS AND ASK THEM TO PALPATE YOUR PERIPHERAL ARTERIAL PULSES AND CHECK THE SENSITIVITY AT YOUR FEET: MONOFILAMENT, VIBRATION, REFLEXES, POSITION, TEMPERATURE AND PRICKS.
> INFORM HIM OF ANY PAIN, HEAT, COLDNESS, SWELLING, PALENESS, REDNESS, BLUE COLOR, PRICKLING SENSATION OR CRAMPS IN THE FEET.

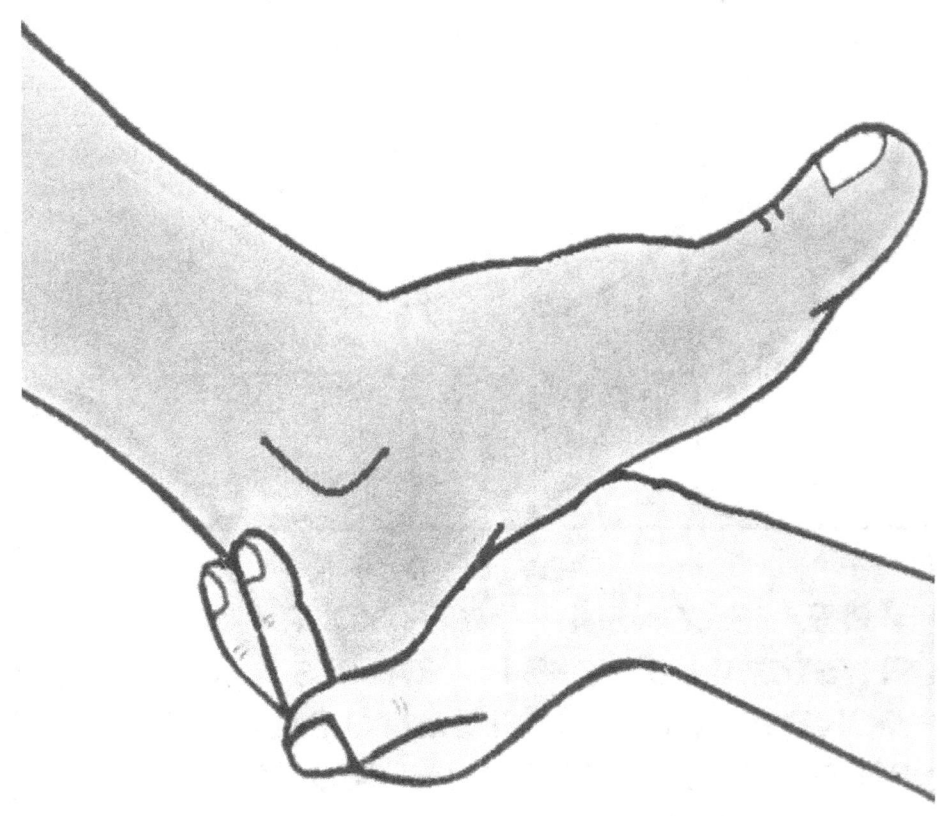

ADVICE #54. CONTINUATION.
REMEMBER THAT YOUR OBJECTIVE IS NOT
ONLY TO DETECT ANY PROBLEM IN THE
FEET, BUT TO REQUEST MEDICAL
ATTENTION FOR ANY COMPLICATION IN
THE LEAST AMOUNT OF TIME.

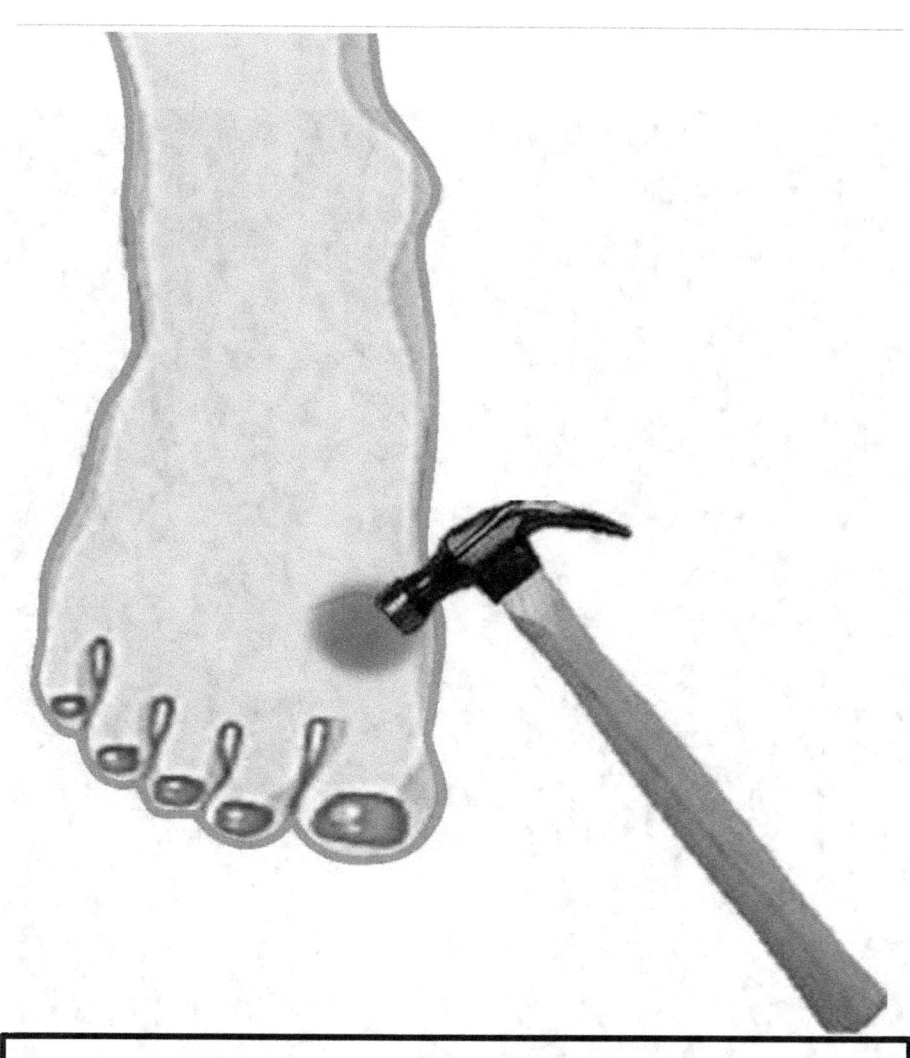

ADVICE #55
> AVOID CONTUSIONS.
SOMETIMES THE COMPLICATIONS OF THE
DIABETIC FOOT ARE TRIGGERED BY A
TRAUMA ON FOOT TISSUE WHICH DO NOT
HAVE SUFFICIENT STRENGTH TO DEFEND
AND RECOVER FROM THE BLOW.

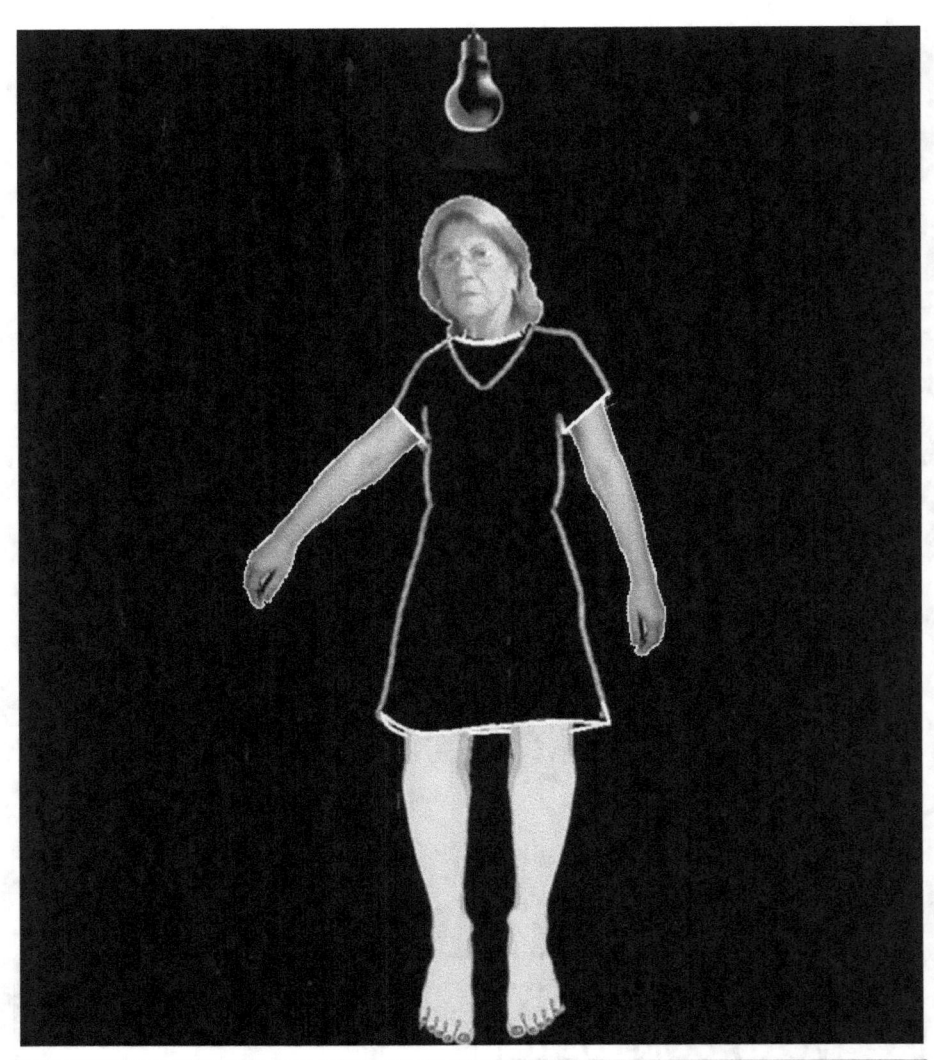

ADVICE #56
> DO NOT WALK IN THE HOUSE WITH THE LIGHTS OFF, BECAUSE YOU CAN RECEIVE A TRAUMA IN YOUR FEET AND START A COMPLICATION.

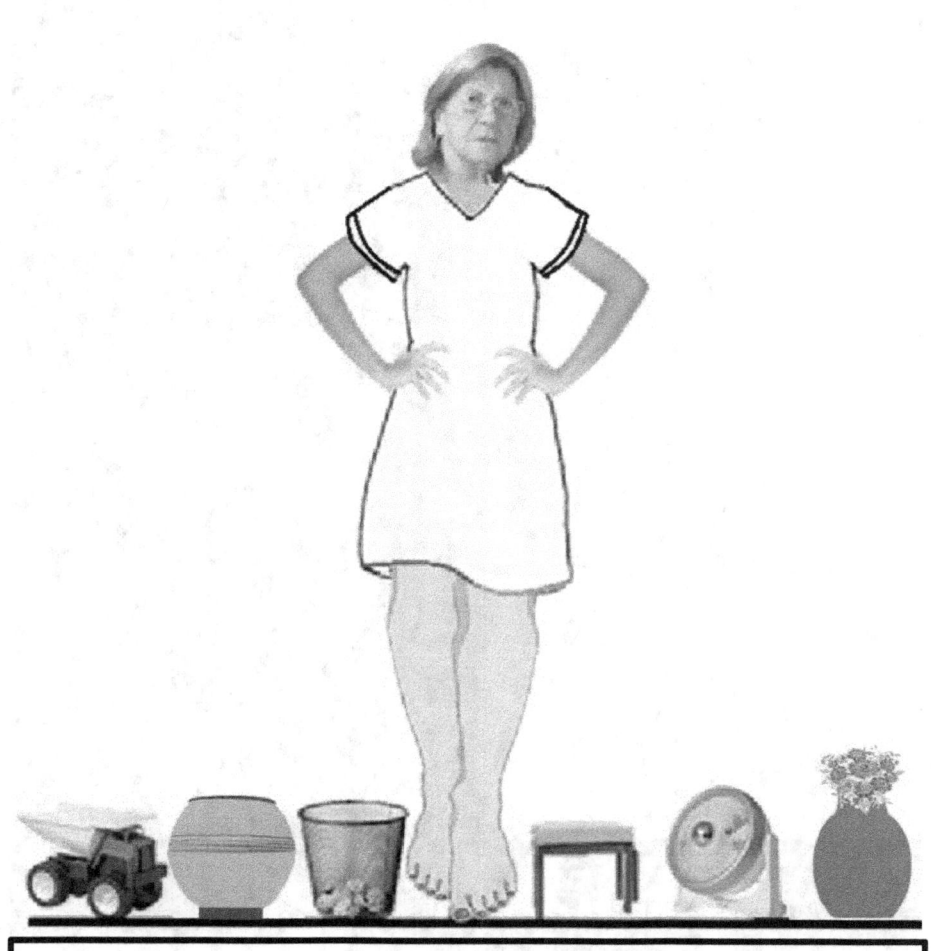

ADVICE #57
DO NOT LEAVE IN THE ROUTE FOR WHICH
YOU WALK IN THE HOUSE SOLID OBJECTS
THAT YOU CAN BUMP INTO THEM WITH
YOUR FEET: FURNITURES, TRASH
BRASSES, VASES, FANS, TOYS, ETC.

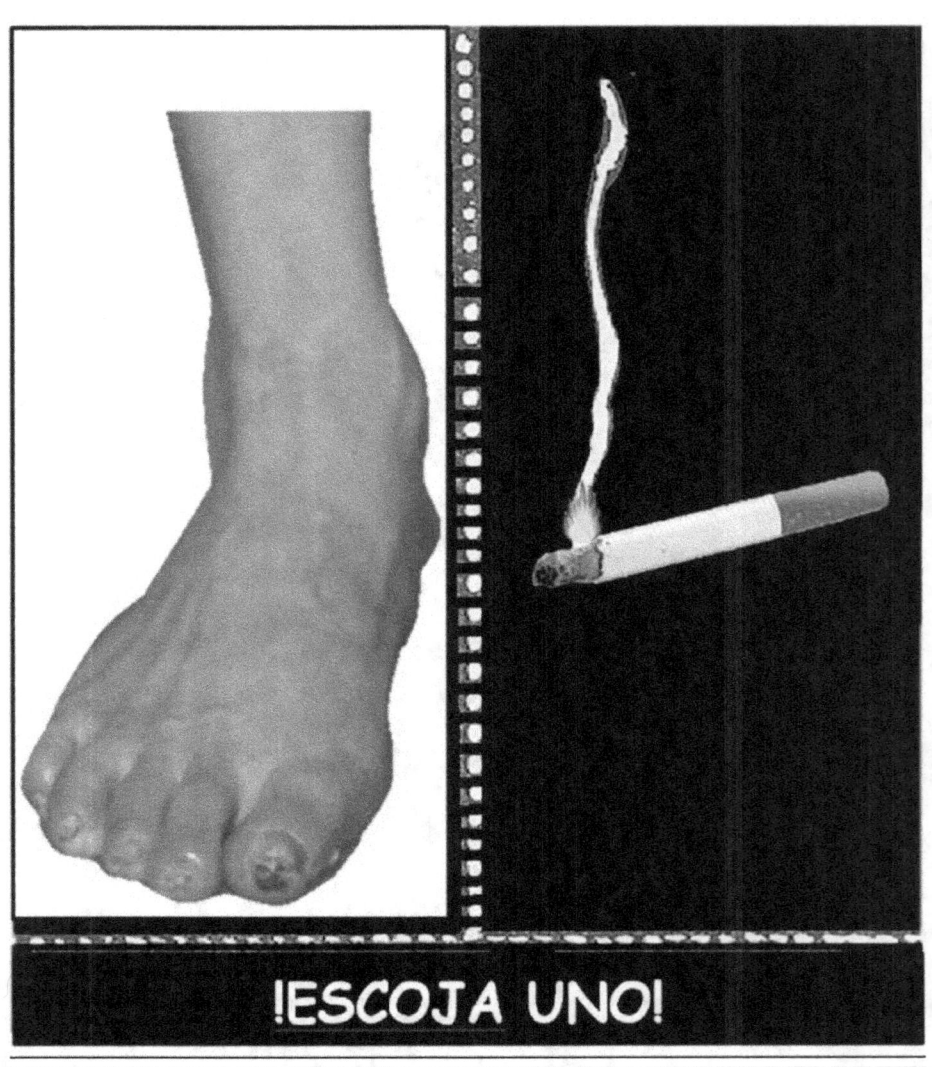

!ESCOJA UNO!

ADVICE #58
DO NOT SMOKE, SMOKING IS HARMFUL TO
THE ARTERIAL CIRCULATION OF DIABETIC
FOOT, FAVORS SPASM AND OCLUSION
(THROMBOSIS) OF THE ARTERIES.

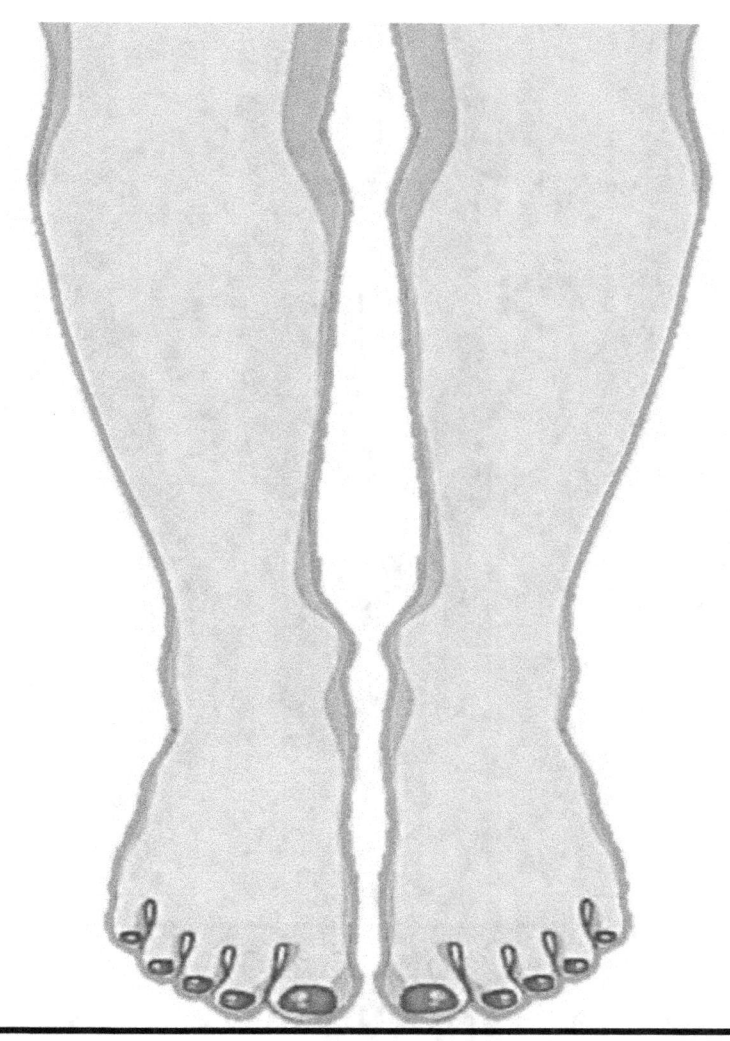

ADVICE #59

BE GENTILE AND LOVING WITH YOUR
FEET. THEY ARE UNDEFENSIVE BEINGS,
THEY PROVIDE AN INVALUABLE SERVICE
TO YOU WITHOUT DEMANDING BENEFITS,
AND THEY DO IT HIDDEN OF THE
EXTERNAL WORLD. BE THANKFUL AND
ALWAYS TRY TO PROTECT THEM.

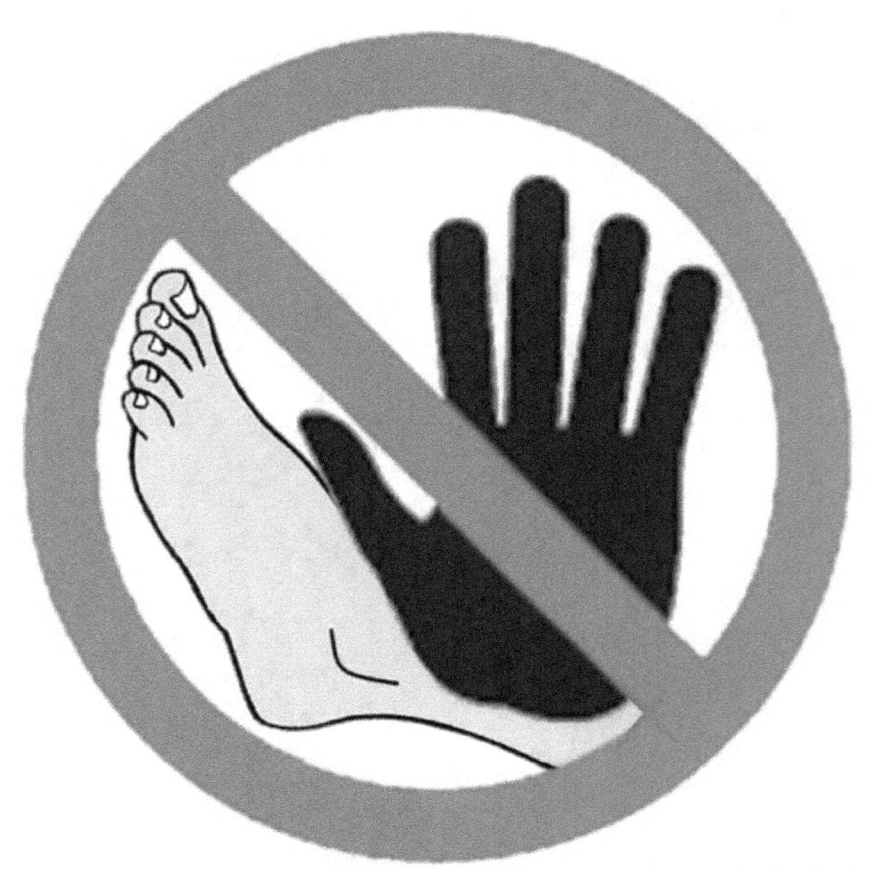

ADVICE #60
DO NOT TAKE ANY INITIATIVE OF YOUR OWN WILL OR BY SUGGESTION OF A FRIEND, WHICH RECOMMENDS APPLYING ANY SUBSTANCE TO THE FEET OR TO CARRY OUT A PROCEDURE WHICH MAY ENDANGER THEIR INTEGRITY, IF IT HAS NOT BEEN CONSULTED AND AUTHORIZED BY YOUR PRIMARY PHYSICIAN OR THE PODIATRIST.

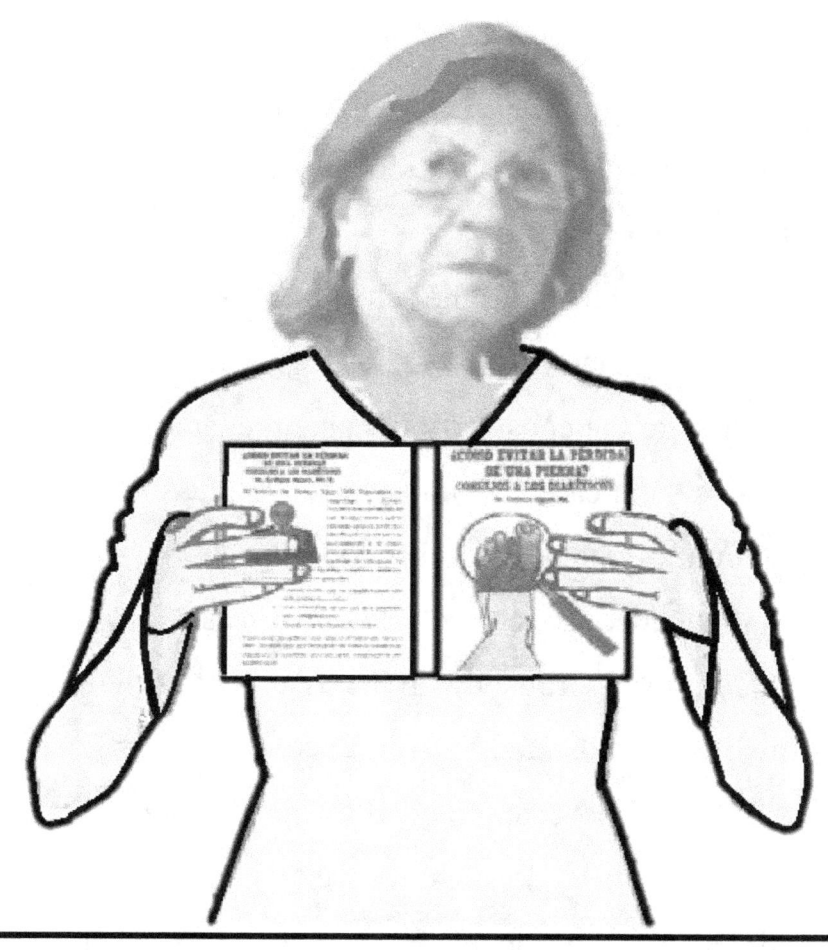

ADVICE #61
PLEASE READ THIS BOOK FRECUENTLY AND
CAREFULLY AND PUT INTO PRACTICE THE
ADVICES IT GIVE TO YOU.
DO NOT FLIP FROM PAGE TO PAGE
OBTAINING ANYTHING, LOOK IN THE
PAGES FOR THE USEFUL KNOWLEDGE THAT
RELEASES YOUR LEGS OF DANGEROUS
COMPLICATIONS.

FINAL SUMMARY

To prevent the complications of your feet, to every diabetic corresponds:

1. Go periodically to the scheduled appointment with your doctor,

2. Prior to the consultation, make the laboratory analysis indicated by your doctor, to measure the amount of glucose in your blood.

3. Take adequate control of your disease:

> Comply rigorously with the treatment of the medicines indicated by your doctor.

> Eat the diet recommended by the dietitian.

> Have your blood sugar tests checked daily, as directed by your doctor.

4, If indicated, do moderate execise

5. Educate yourself to master the basic knowledge of diabetes.

6. Read this book from time to time and follow its advice.

7. Going to educational activities imparted by your Health Plan about "Diabetic Foot Care".

8. Avoid by all means trauma to your feet.

9. Be careful in the selection of shoes to use.

10. Examine your feet periodically.

11. Distract yourself.

12. Stay at your normal weight.

13. Do not smoke!

And remember, diabetic patient, that your goal in accepting and carrying out these advices is to avoid an amputation in your legs.

BIBLIOGRAPHY

1. Age-Adjusted Hospital Discharge Rates for Nontraumatic Lower Extremity Amputation per 1000 Diabetic Population, by Sex. United States, 1993-2002. Atlanta, CA: Center for Disease Control and Prevention; National Center for Chronic Disease Prevention and Health.

2. Age-Adjusted Hospital Discharge Rates for Nontraumatic Lower Extremity Amputation per 1000 Diabetic Population, by Level of Amputation, United States, 1993-2002. Atlanta, CA: Center for Disease Control and Prevention; National Center for Chronic Disease Prevention and Health.

3. Age-Adjusted Hospital Discharge Rates for Nontraumatic Lower Extremity Amputation per 1000 Diabetic Population, by Race, United States, 1993-2002. Atlanta, CA: Center for Disease Control and Prevention; National Center for Chronic Disease Prevention and Health.

4. Ahroni, Jessie H. PhD, 101 Foot Care Tips for People with Diabetes. American Diabetes Association. 2000.

5. Bakker, K. Riley, P. El año del pie diabético. Diabetes'Voice.2005. Vol. 50, No1.

6. Boulton, A. JM; Connor, H. and Cavanagh, P. The Foot in Diabetes. John Wiley & Sons Ltd. 2000.

7. Claud, Linda. Diabetes Foot Cure: Tips To Save Your Foot. Ju8n 1, 2015. Kindle Edition.

8. Dutton, Elizabeth. Essential Foot Care for Diabetics (Foot Care for You Series from The Foot Care Center) Book 1. Mar 16, 2012. Kindle Edition.

9. Fielding, JE. Smoking health effects and control. N. Engl. J. Med. 1985; 31:491-498.

10. Gillen, C. et all. There Is A Hole in My Foot: A guide to diabetic foot ulcers. May 9, 2016. Kindle edition.

11. Hogan, P. et al. Economic Costs of Diabetes in USA in 2002. Diabetes Care 26. 2003. 917-32.

12. Krupski, W.C. The peripheral vascular consequences of smoking. Amm. Vasc. Surg;5:291-304.

13. Menzoin, J.O. et all. Symptomatology and anatomic patterns of peripheral vascular disease; different impact of smoking and diabetes. Ann. Vasc. Surg. 1989;3:224-228.

14. Malone, J, M. et all, Prevention of amputation by diabetic education. Am J Surg. 1989.

15. National Diabetes Statistics Report. 2014. Center for Disease Control.

16. Organización Mundial de la Salud. Reporte. 2014

17. Owings, M., Kozak LJ. National Center for Health S. Ambulatory and Inpatient Procedures in the United States, 1996. Hyattsville, Md.: U.S. Dept. of Health and Human Services, Centers for Disease Control and Prevention, National Center for Health Statistics; 1998. (2)

18. Pandian, G., et all. Rehabilitation of the Patient with Peripheral Vascular Disease and Diabetic Foot Problems. In: DeLisa JA, Gans BM, editors. Philadelphia: Lippincott-Raven; 1998. (6).

19. Pie Diabético. Epidemiología. Wounds International. 2013.

20. Ruderman, N., Devlin, J.T., Eds. Health Professional's Guide to Diabetes and Exercise. American Diabetes Association. Alexandria. VA. 1996.

21. Scheffler, N. M. DPM, FACFAS. 21 Things you need to know about diabetes and your feet. American Diabetic Association. 2012.

22. Sidawy, A.N. Diabetic Foot Lower Extremity Arterial Disease and Limb Salvage. Lippincott Williams & Wilkins. 2006.

23. Swidorski, D. e t all. Foot Care (Defeat Rules for Survival).21, 2013. Kindle Edition.

INDEX

Introduction. 1.

Complications of the Arterial Blood Circulation by Reduction or Absence of Blood (Ischemic). 4.

Infectious Complications for Penetration and Development of Germs. 8.

Complications due to Nerve Damage (Diabetic Neuropathy). 10.

Joints Complications. (Deformities). 11.

The feet Exam. 13.

Advices for Diabetics Patients to Avoid Leg Amputation. 15.

Final Summary. 92.

Bibliography. 94.

OF THE AUTHOR

Professor Dr. Enrique Uguet PhD Specialist in Angiology and Vascular Surgery, has accumulated a vast experience in the diagnosis and treatment of complications of diabetic foot, having treated hundreds of them, by means of medicines administered orally, intramuscularly, intravenously and intrarterial.

He has performed revascularization surgery: thrombo-endarterectomies, venous patches, autogenous venous grafts, plastics: aortoiliac, femoro-popliteal, skin, lumbar gangliectomies, debridements, incisions and drainage.

Locally in compress and in footbaths has used: potassium permanganate, hydrogen peroxide, placentotherapy, antibiotic ointments, nitrofurazone, growth factor and in a considerable number of occasions the hyperbaric chamber. And when it has been necessary, to save part of a limb, he has been in the inescapable need to carry out a minor amputation, or to preserve the patient's life, a greater amputation.

He has also performed surgical procedures for abdominal aortic aneurysms, carotid arteries, erectile dysfunction and varicose veins.

He is the author of numerous scientific publications in national and international journals and books such as: Acute Deep Thrombophlebitis of Lower Limbs, Advice to Diabetic Patients. Care of their Feet, How the Students' Brain Learn, and Theory of Labor Stability of Teachers through Natural School Selection.

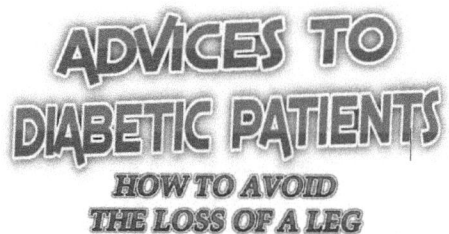

ADVICES TO DIABETIC PATIENTS

HOW TO AVOID
THE LOSS OF A LEG

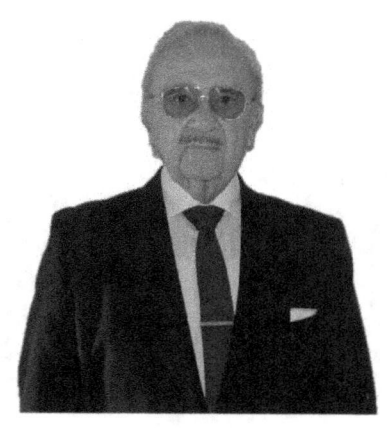

Professor Dr. Enrique Uguet PhD Specialist in Angiology and Vascular Surgery is convinced that the best way for diabetics to avoid a complication in their feet is to prevent it and the most appropriate way to avoid it is through education, which must incorporate as a totem or protective emblem, which is based on three general principles:

1. Know the complications that may happen to them.

2. Be aware of why these complications occur.

3. And what are the ways to avoid them.

Towards these three pillars, the contents of this book are designed to obtain from the reader the strength of conscience and conduct necessary to fulfill these advices in their daily life.